DIABETIC RENAL DIET COOKBOOK FOR NEWLY DIAGNOSED 2024

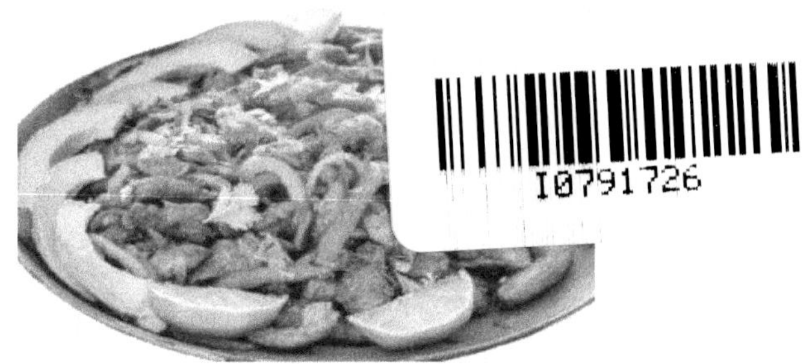

The Ultimate Guide to Managing Diabetes and Kidney Disease for Newly Diagnosed

BETTY J. BAKKE

TABLE OF CONTENT

4

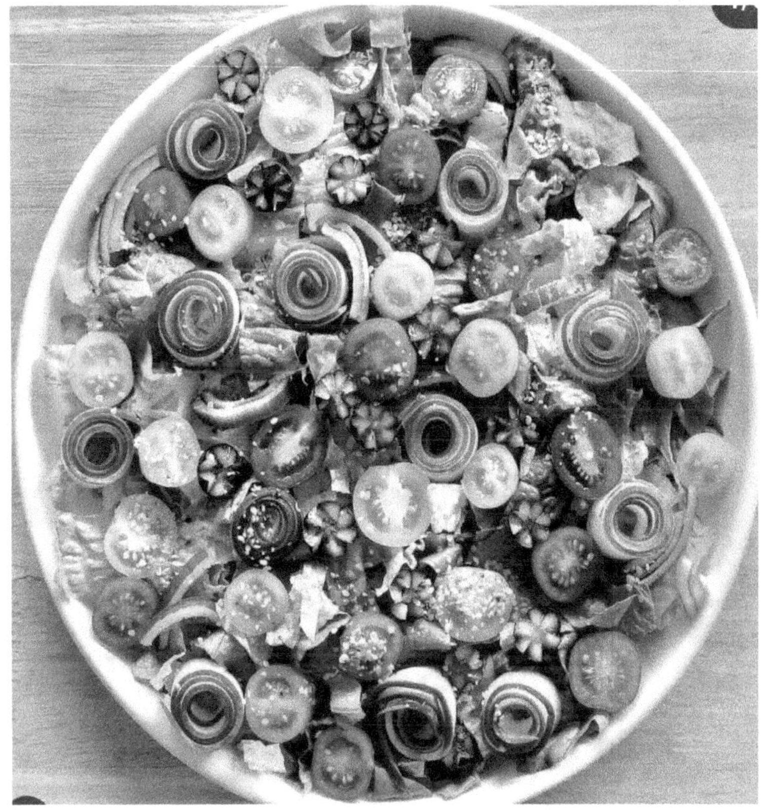

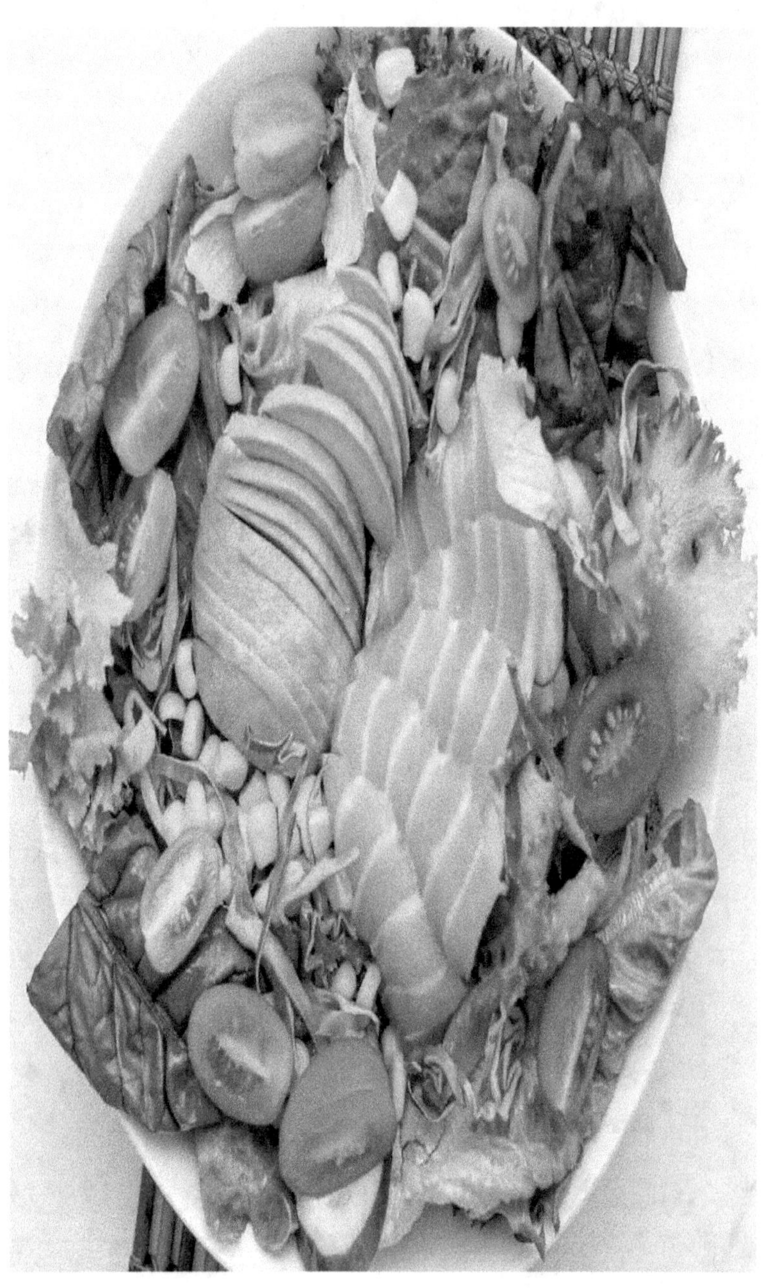

INTRODUCTION

It can be difficult to deal with a diabetes diagnosis and kidney problems, particularly for people starting a new chapter in their health journey. In 2024, we need to work toward better healthcare and a deeper comprehension of nutritional control, therefore it's critical to offer specialized assistance to individuals juggling these two competing demands. For a person who have just received a diagnosis and are starting their diabetic renal diet, this introduction provides guidance.

As we explore the nuances of co-managing these two illnesses, it is imperative to acknowledge the significant influence that diet can have on overall health consequences. This cookbook is more than simply a list of recipes; it's an all-inclusive guide meant to provide people the information and resources they need to make wise dietary decisions.

This cookbook provides newly diagnosed patients with practical counsel, delectable recipes, and useful insights into creating a balanced and nutritious diet. From comprehending the necessity of portion control to learning how to include nutrient-dense products, every facet of dietary management is handled with care and compassion.

By adopting the concepts of a diabetic renal diet, a patients may take proactive actions to improve their health and well-being. They can improve their quality of life and better manage their conditions by making simple modifications to their food habits and lifestyle.

In the pulsating metropolis of 2024, despite the continual hum of technology progress and medical discoveries, there is a quiet nook where the lives of newly diagnosed people collide with the delicate balance between health and diet. In the core of this story, we meet a diverse ensemble of characters: people who have recently gotten the difficult diagnosis of diabetes and kidney difficulties.

Among them is Mrs. Thompson, a lively Aunt with a passion for cooking who is now left with the onerous challenge of reinventing her favorite dishes to meet her new dietary constraints. Then there's Mr. Patel, an engineer who takes pleasure in his independence but suddenly finds himself navigating a tangle of dietary recommendations and medical advice.

As these people deal with their illnesses, they become drawn to a common thread: the diabetic renal diet. In this first installment of their trip, we follow them as they seek information and insight, as well as the tools and resources they will require to navigate this new chapter in their lives.

Together, they discover the secrets of balanced nutrition and learn how to manage their diseases via mindful eating and good lifestyle choices. Along the process, they learn the value of community and support, finding strength in one another as they confront the obstacles that lie ahead.

As their journey progresses, we are reminded of the strength of the human spirit and the transformational power of knowledge. So, with courage in their hearts and resolve in their eyes, our characters go on a path of recovery and hope, led by diabetic renal diet principles and the promise of a better tomorrow.

1. Chicken salad

Ingredients:

2 cups cooked chicken breast, diced or shredded

1/2 cup celery, finely chopped

1/4 cup red onion, finely chopped

1/4 cup grapes, halved

1/4 cup almonds, sliced

1/4 cup Greek yogurt

2 tablespoons mayonnaise

1 tablespoon lemon juice

1 teaspoon Dijon mustard

Salt and black pepper to taste

Preparation: In a large mixing bowl, add diced or shredded chicken breast, celery, red onion, grapes, and almonds. In a small mixing bowl, combine the Greek yogurt, mayonnaise, lemon juice, Dijon mustard, salt, and black pepper until thoroughly blended. Toss the dressing into the chicken mixture until evenly covered. Taste and adjust seasoning as needed. Cover the bowl and chill the chicken salad for at least 30 minutes to enable the flavors to combine.

Nutritional Value (per serving, approximately 1 cup):

Calories: 250 kcal

Protein: 25g

Fat: 12g

Carbohydrates: 10g

Fiber: 2g

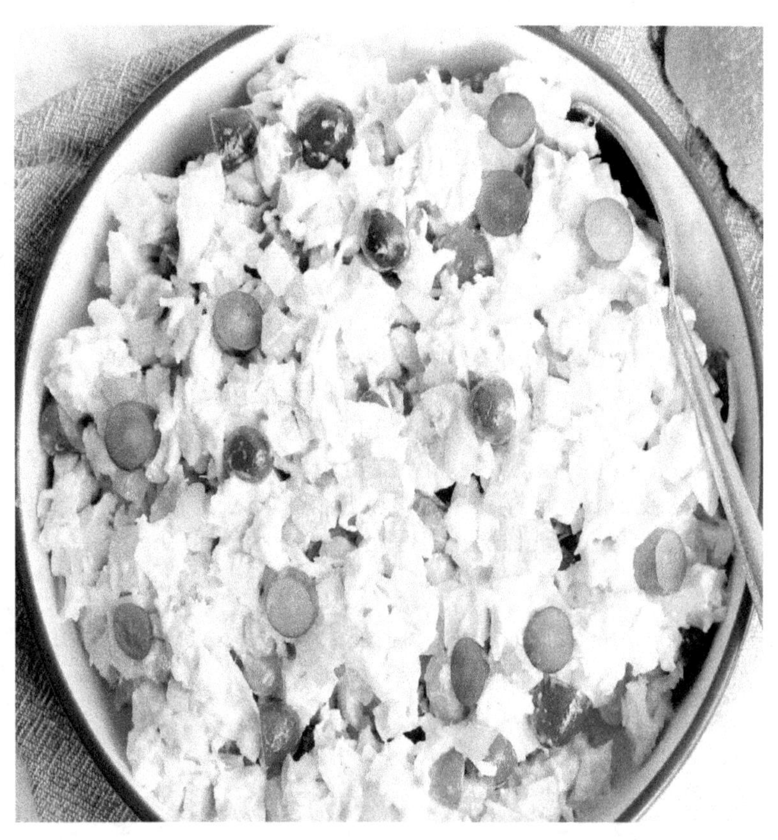

2.Baked Apples with Crumble Topping

Ingredients:

4 large apples (such as Granny Smith or Honeycrisp)

1/4 cup rolled oats

2 tablespoons all-purpose flour

2 tablespoons brown sugar (or sweetener of choice)

2 tablespoons unsalted butter, chilled and cubed

1/4 teaspoon ground cinnamon

Pinch of salt

Vanilla ice cream or whipped cream for serving (optional)

Preparation: Preheat the oven to 375°F (190° C). Lightly grease or line a baking dish with parchment paper. Wash the apples, then remove the cores using an apple corer or a knife, leaving the bottoms intact to form a hole. In a bowl, combine the rolled oats, all-purpose flour, brown sugar, cooled butter cubes, ground cinnamon, and a pinch of salt. Using your fingers or a fork, combine the ingredients until they resemble coarse crumbs. Fill each cored apple with the crumble mixture, pressing gently into the well. Bake the filled apples in the preheated oven for 25-30 minutes, or until the apples are cooked and the crumble topping has turned golden brown.

Nutritional Value (per serving, one baked apple):

Calories: 200 kcal

Protein: 2g

11

Fat: 8g

Carbohydrates: 35g

Fiber: 5g

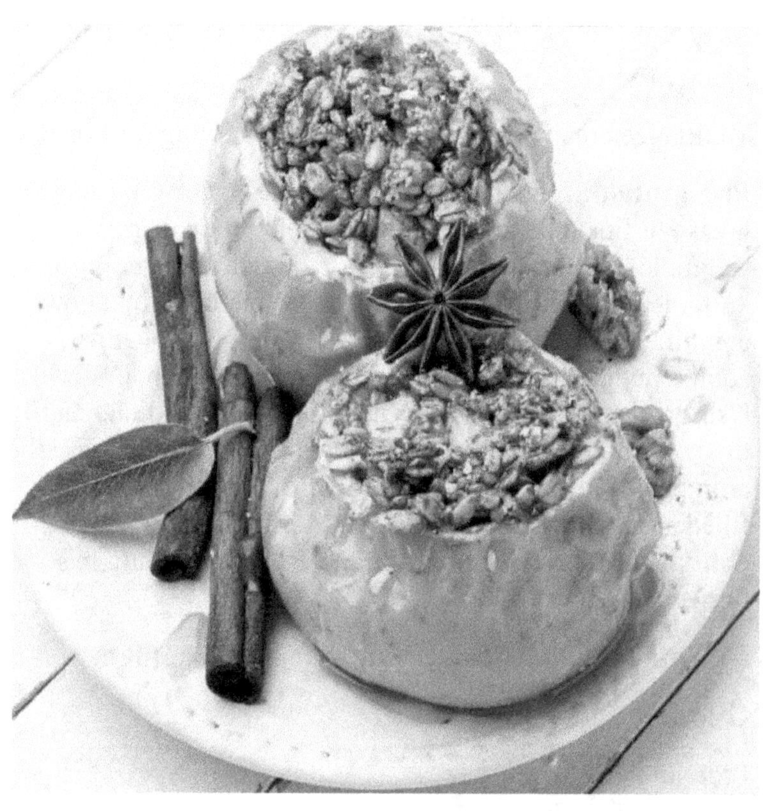

3.Pumpkin-Free Pumpkin Pie

Ingredients:

Graham cracker crumbs

Sugar

Butter

Sweet potato puree

Butternut squash puree

Brown sugar

Maple syrup

Eggs

Heavy cream

Vanilla extract, spices.

Preparation: To make the crust, combine graham cracker crumbs, sugar, and melted butter. Press into a pie plate. Combine sweet potato puree, butternut squash puree, sugar, eggs, cream, and spices; pour into the crust. Bake until completely set. Allow pie to cool completely before slicing. If preferred, serve with whipped cream or ice cream.

Nutritional Value (for 8 serving)

Calories: 350-400 kcal

Protein: 5-7g

Fat: 20-25g

Carbohydrates: 35-40g

Fiber:2-3g

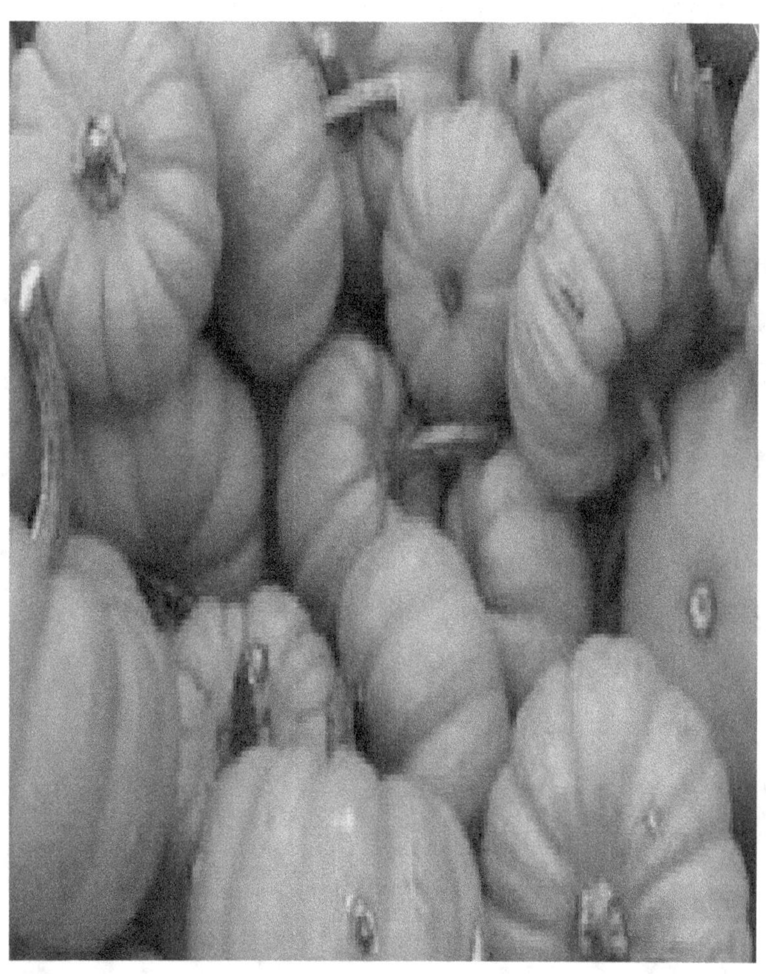

4.Creamy Spinach Couscous Risotto

Ingredients:

1 cup couscous

2 cups vegetable or chicken broth

1 tablespoon olive oil

1 small onion, finely chopped

2 cloves garlic, minced

2 cups fresh spinach, chopped

1/2 cup grated Parmesan cheese

1/4 cup heavy cream

Salt and pepper to taste

Preparation: Begin by cooking couscous in a delicious broth to enhance its richness. Sauté the onion and garlic until fragrant, filling the dish with rich flavor. Gradually add the heated broth, stirring until the couscous is creamy. Add fresh spinach, enabling its brilliant color to brighten the meal. After removing from heat, add grated Parmesan and rich heavy cream to improve the texture and taste profile. Season to your liking.

Nutritional value (per serving, approximately 1 cup):

Calories: 250 kcal

Protein: 9g

Fat: 10g

Carbohydrates: 30g

Fiber: 3g

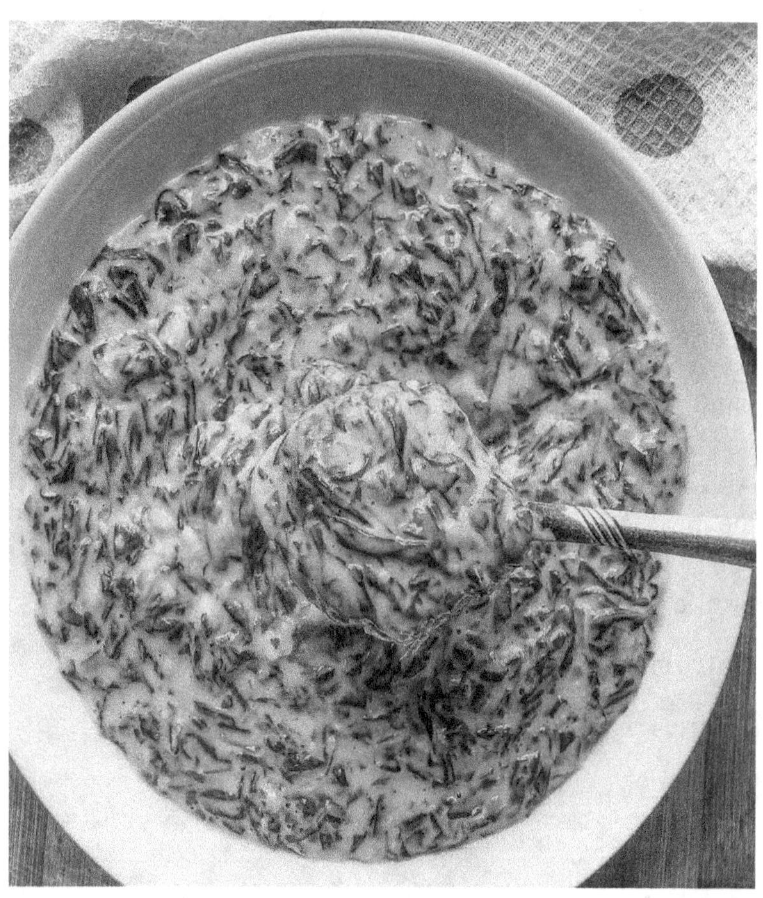

5.Apple and Peanut Butter

Ingredients:

1 medium-sized apple (any variety you prefer)

2 tablespoons peanut butter (smooth or crunchy, as per your preference)

Preparation: Wash the apple thoroughly under running water, then wipe it dry with a clean kitchen towel. Core the apple and slice it into tiny wedges or rounds, whichever you choose. Place the apple slices on a serving dish or a cutting board, arranged neatly. Scoop the peanut butter onto the dish beside the apple slices, or straight onto each slice if you like. Serve immediately and enjoy!

Nutritional value per serving of apple and peanut butter (based on one medium-sized apple and two tablespoons of peanut butter):

Calories: 285 kcal

Protein: 7 grams

Fat: 16 grams

Carbohydrates: 31 grams

Fiber: 5 grams

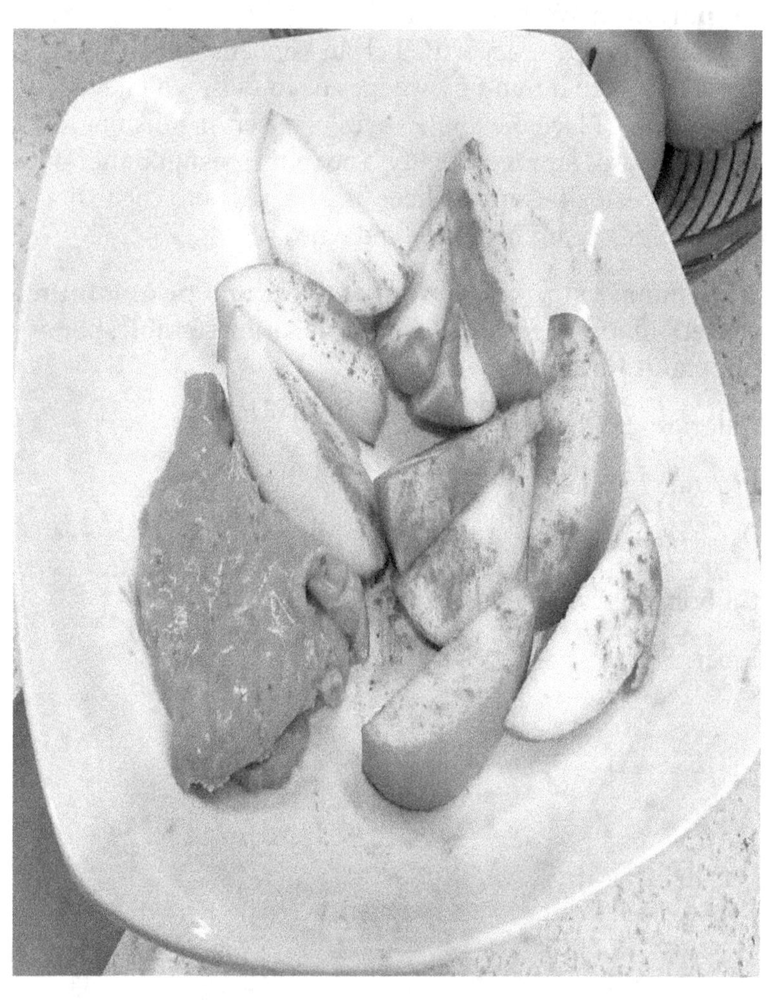

6.Masala Omelet with Mixed Veggies

Ingredients:

2 large eggs

1/4 cup mixed vegetables (such as bell peppers, onions, tomatoes, spinach, mushrooms, etc.), finely chopped

1 green chili, finely chopped (optional)

1 tablespoon chopped cilantro (coriander leaves)

1/4 teaspoon turmeric powder

1/4 teaspoon cumin powder

1/4 teaspoon chili powder (adjust to taste)

Salt, 1 tablespoon oil or butter, for cooking

Preparation: In a mixing basin, beat the eggs until completely combined. Mix in the mixed veggies, green chili (if using), chopped cilantro, turmeric powder, cumin powder, chili powder, and salt to the beaten eggs. Mix everything together until well blended. Heat oil or butter in a nonstick pan over medium heat. Pour the egg and vegetable mixture into the skillet and distribute evenly to coat the bottom. Cook the omelet for 2-3 minutes, or until the bottom is set and gently browned. Carefully turn the omelet with a spatula and cook for another 2-3 minutes on the other side, or until thoroughly done.

Nutritional Value per serving (approximately one omelet):

Calories: 200 kcal

Protein: 12 grams

Fat:14 grams

Carbohydrates: 5 grams

Fiber: 1.5 grams

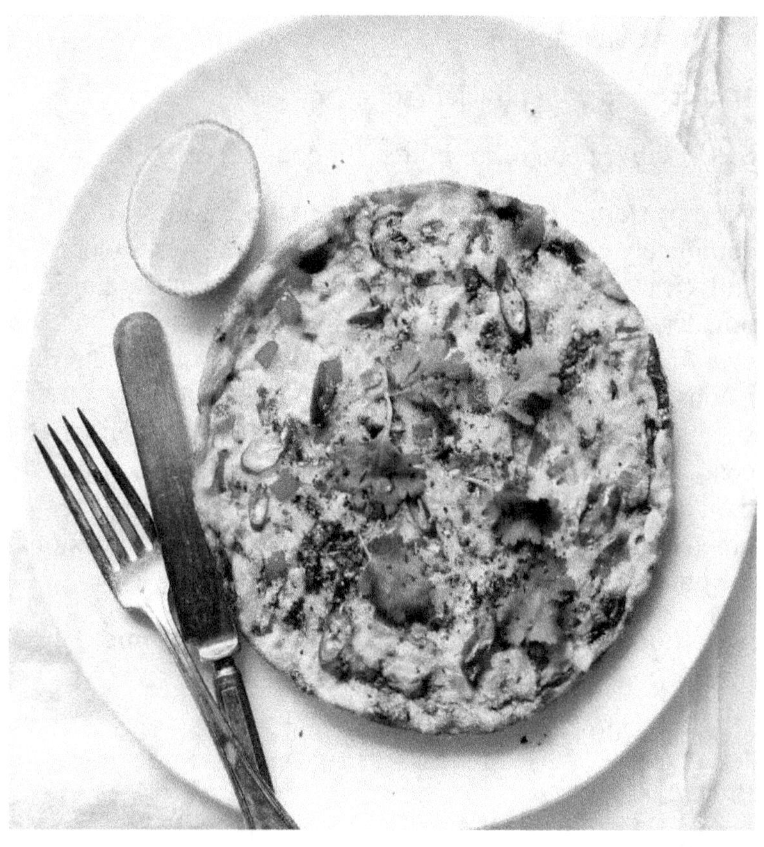

7.Pesto

Ingredients:

2 cups fresh basil leaves, packed

1/4 cup pine nuts or walnuts

1/4 cup grated Parmesan cheese

2 cloves garlic, peeled

1/2 cup extra virgin olive oil

Salt and pepper, to taste

Preparation Method: In a food processor or blender, mix fresh basil leaves, pine nuts or walnuts, grated Parmesan cheese, and peeled garlic cloves. Pulse the ingredients a few times until coarsely chopped. With the food processor or blender running, gently sprinkle in the olive oil until the pesto achieves the desired consistency. You may need to pause and scrape down the bowl's sides as needed. Season the pesto with salt and pepper, to taste. Blend briefly to integrate. Once the pesto has reached the proper consistency and taste, transfer it to a clean jar or container to store.

Nutritional Value per serving (approximately 2 tablespoons):

Calories: 120 kcal

Protein: 2 grams

Fat: 12 grams

Carbohydrates: 1 gram

Fiber: 0.5 grams

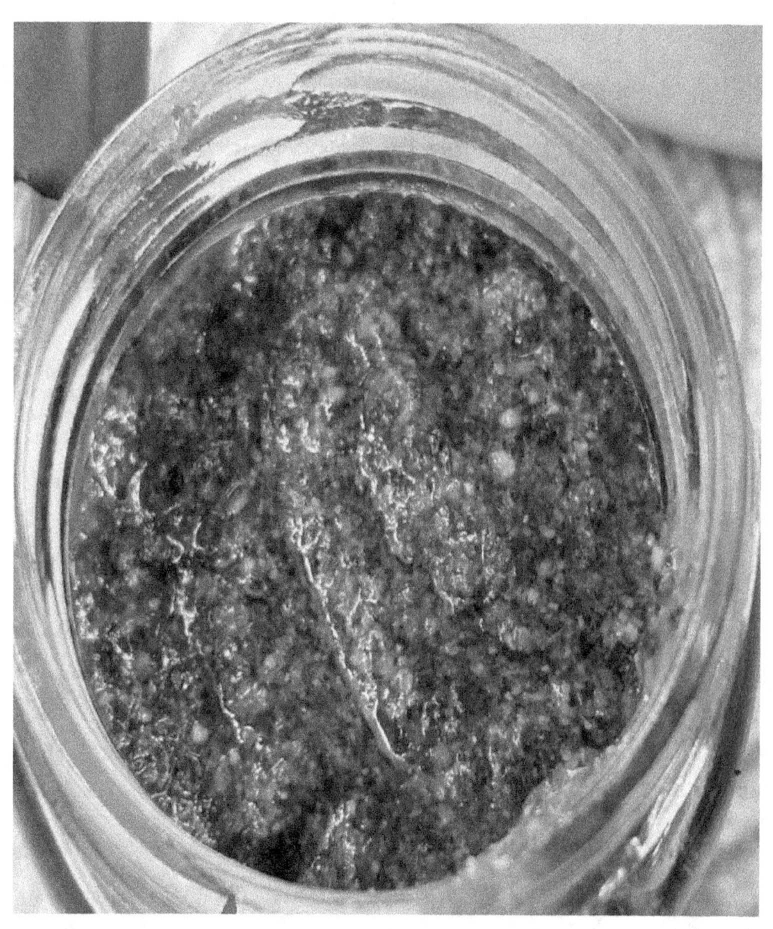

8.Wild Rice Mushroom Soup

Ingredients:

1 cup wild rice, 8 cups vegetable or chicken broth

2 tablespoons olive oil or butter

1 onion, finely chopped, 2 cloves garlic, minced

8 ounces mushrooms (such as cremini or white button), sliced

1 carrot, 1 celery stalk, diced, 1/4 cup all-purpose flour

2 cups milk (or dairy-free alternative)

1/2 cup heavy cream (optional)

Salt and pepper, to taste

Fresh parsley or thyme, for garnish (optional)

Preparation: Prepare the wild rice by simmering it gently in flavorful broth until tender. Sauté a medley of aromatic ingredients including onion, garlic, mushrooms, carrot, and celery until they release their rich flavors. Incorporate a roux made with flour to thicken the soup, then gradually introduce creamy milk and optionally indulgent heavy cream for added richness. Allow the soup to simmer gently, marrying the flavors beautifully as it cooks with the tender wild rice. Finish with a sprinkle of fresh parsley for a burst of color and freshness.

Nutritional Value per serving (approximately 1 cup):

Calories: 200 kcal

Protein: 7 grams

Fat: 8 grams

Carbohydrates: 28 grams

Fiber: 3 grams

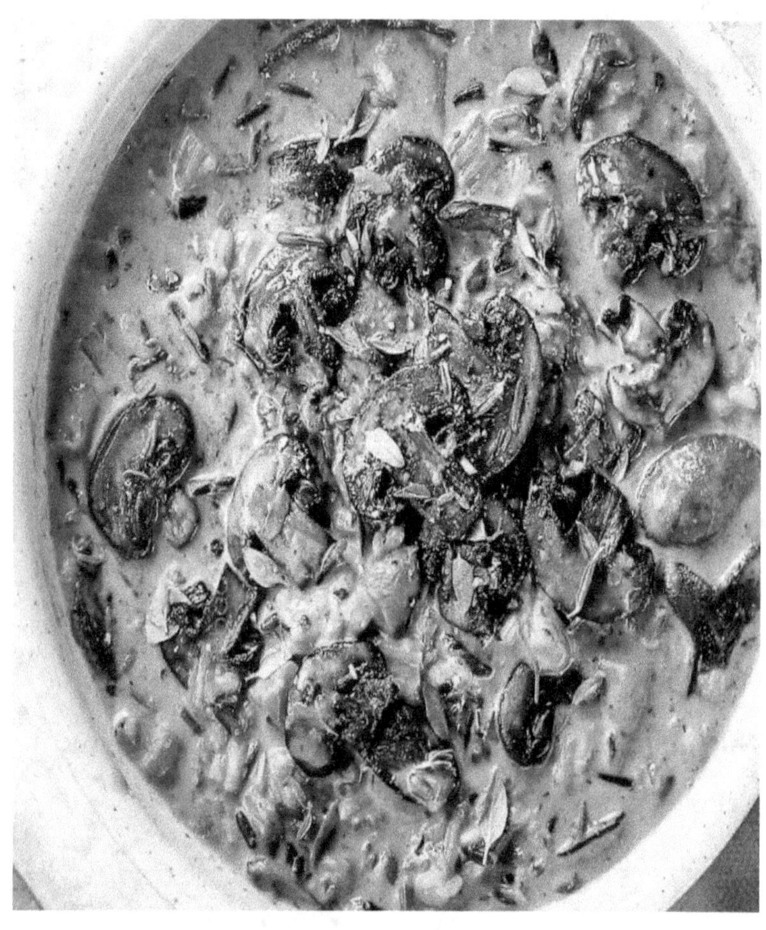

9.Quibebe Soup

Ingredients:

1 medium-sized butternut squash, peeled, seeded, and diced

1 onion, finely chopped

2 cloves garlic, minced

1 bell pepper,1 tomato,1 carrot,1 celery stalk, diced

1 cup corn kernels (fresh, frozen, or canned)

1 cup cooked black beans

4 cups vegetable broth

2 tablespoons olive oil

1 teaspoon cumin,1 teaspoon paprika

Salt and pepper, to taste

Fresh cilantro, chopped, for garnish

Preparation: Begin by sautéing aromatic onion, garlic, and bell pepper until fragrant. Then, incorporate a vibrant array of vegetables including tomato, carrot, celery, squash, corn, and black beans. Season generously with warming spices like cumin and paprika, along with a pinch of salt and pepper. Simmer the medley in nourishing vegetable broth until the squash is tender, allowing the flavors to meld. Before serving, garnish with a sprinkle of fresh cilantro for a burst of freshness. Adjust the ingredients and seasoning to suit personal preferences.

Nutritional Value per serving (approximately 1 cup):

Calories: 50 kcal

Protein: 5 grams

Fat: 5 grams

Carbohydrates: 25 grams

Fiber: 6 grams

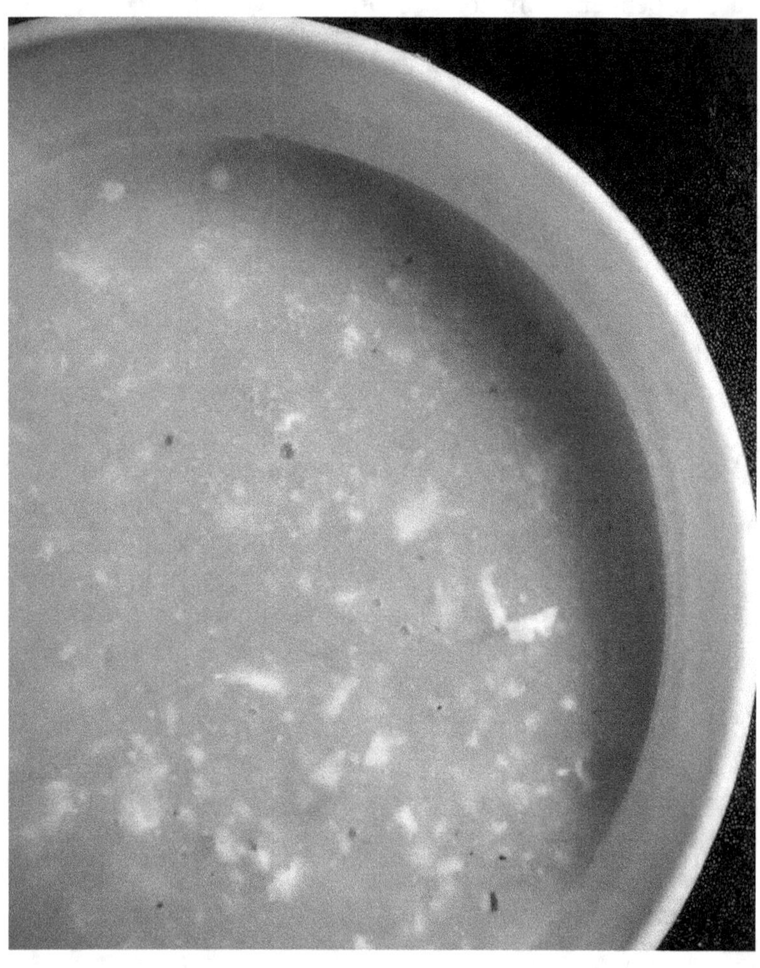

10.Low Sodium Chicken Stock

Ingredients:

2 lbs chicken bones or carcasses

2 onions, quartered

2 carrots, chopped

2 celery stalks, chopped

2 cloves garlic, smashed

2 bay leaves

1 tablespoon whole peppercorns

Handful of fresh parsley

Water

Preparation: In a large stockpot, combine chicken bones, onions, carrots, celery, garlic, bay leaves, peppercorns, and parsley. Fill the saucepan with water until the contents are completely immersed. Bring to a boil, then reduce heat to low and simmer uncovered for 3-4 hours, skimming any impurities that rise to the surface. Strain the stock through a fine mesh sieve and let it cool before storing in containers.

Nutritional Value:

Calories: 15 kcal

Protein: 1g

Fat: 0g

Carbohydrates: 1g

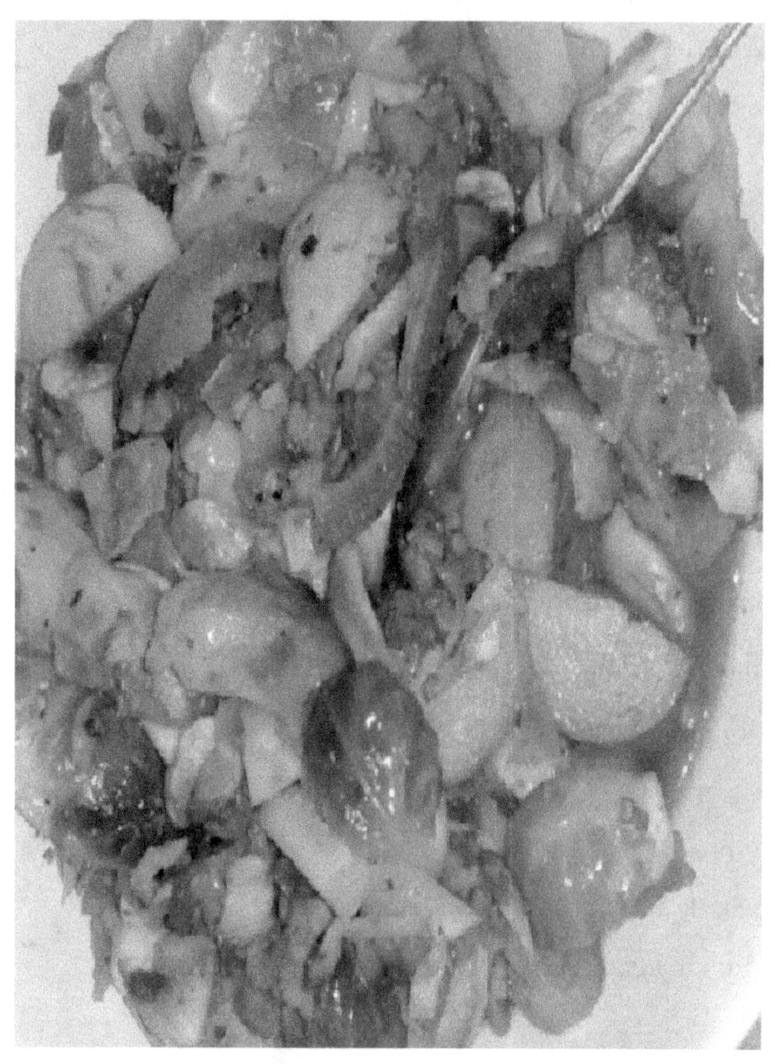

11. Gingery Chicken Noodle Soup

Ingredients:

6 cups low sodium chicken stock (prepared from above)

2 boneless, skinless chicken breasts

2-inch piece ginger, thinly sliced

2 cloves garlic, minced

2 carrots, thinly sliced

2 celery stalks, thinly sliced

4 oz rice noodles

Salt and pepper to taste

Fresh cilantro, chopped, for garnish

Preparation Method: In a large saucepan, bring chicken stock to a simmer. Combine chicken breasts, ginger, and garlic. Simmer for 15-20 minutes, or until the chicken is well cooked. Remove the chicken from the saucepan and shred using forks. Return shredded chicken to the pot. Add carrots and celery to the pot and simmer until vegetables are tender, about 10 minutes. Meanwhile, cook rice noodles according to package instructions. Drain and set aside. Add cooked noodles to the soup. Season with salt and pepper to taste.

Nutritional Value:

Calories: 250 kcal

Protein: 20g

Fat: 3g

Carbohydrates: 35g

Fiber: 2g

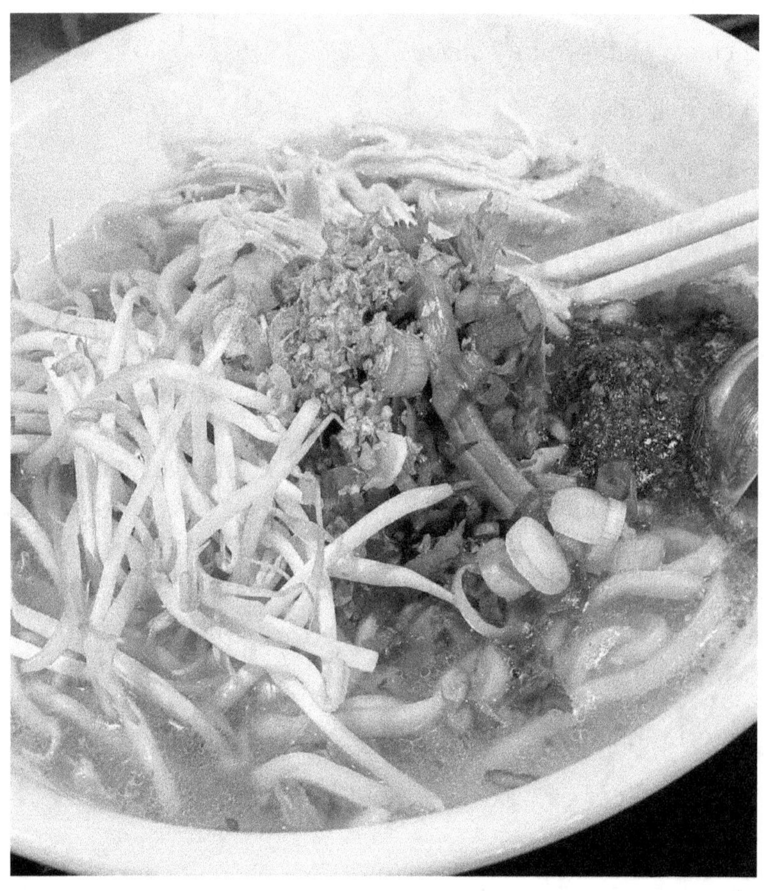

12. Fire Roasted Corn Soup

Ingredients:

4 cups fire-roasted corn kernels

1 onion, chopped

2 cloves garlic, minced

4 cups low sodium chicken stock (prepared from above)

1 cup heavy cream

Salt and pepper to taste

Fresh chives, chopped, for garnish

Preparation: In a large saucepan, sauté the onions and garlic until softened. Add the fire-roasted corn kernels and the chicken stock to the saucepan. Simmer for 15-20 minutes. To make the soup smooth, use an immersion blender. Alternatively, transfer the soup to a blender in stages and process until smooth before returning it to the saucepan. Stir in the heavy cream and cook for a further 5 minutes. Add salt and pepper to taste. Serve hot, topped with fresh chives.

Nutritional Value:

Calories: 200 kcal

Protein: 4g

Fat: 12g

Carbohydrates: 20g

Fiber: 2g

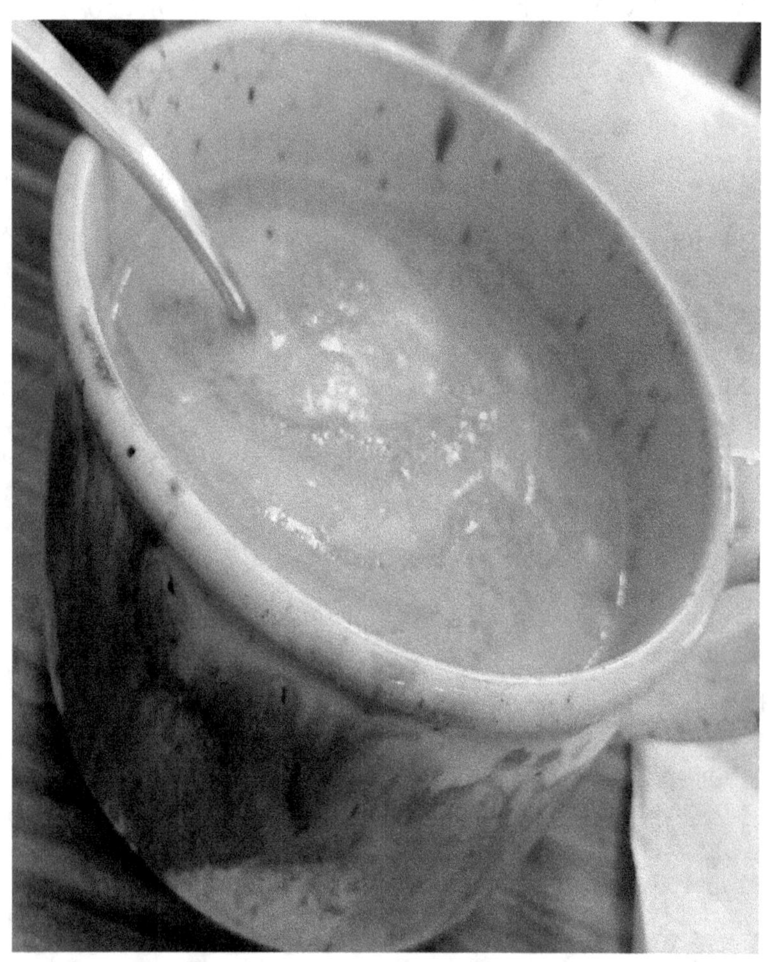

13. Baked Apples with Cherries and Almonds

Ingredients:

4 apples, cored

1/2 cup dried cherries

1/4 cup slivered almonds

1/4 cup brown sugar or sweetener of choice

1 teaspoon ground cinnamon

1/4 teaspoon ground nutmeg

1/4 cup water

Vanilla ice cream or whipped cream, for serving (optional)

Preparation: Preheat oven to 375°F (190°C). In a bowl, mix together dried cherries, slivered almonds, brown sugar, cinnamon, and nutmeg. Stuff each cored apple with the cherry-almond mixture. Place stuffed apples in a baking dish and pour water into the bottom of the dish. Cover with foil and bake for 30-40 minutes, until apples are soft. Serve warm, with the option of topping with vanilla ice cream or whipped cream.

Nutritional Value:

Calories: 150 kcal (per apple)

Protein: 2g

Fat: 4g

Carbohydrates: 30g

Fiber: 5g

Sugar: 20g

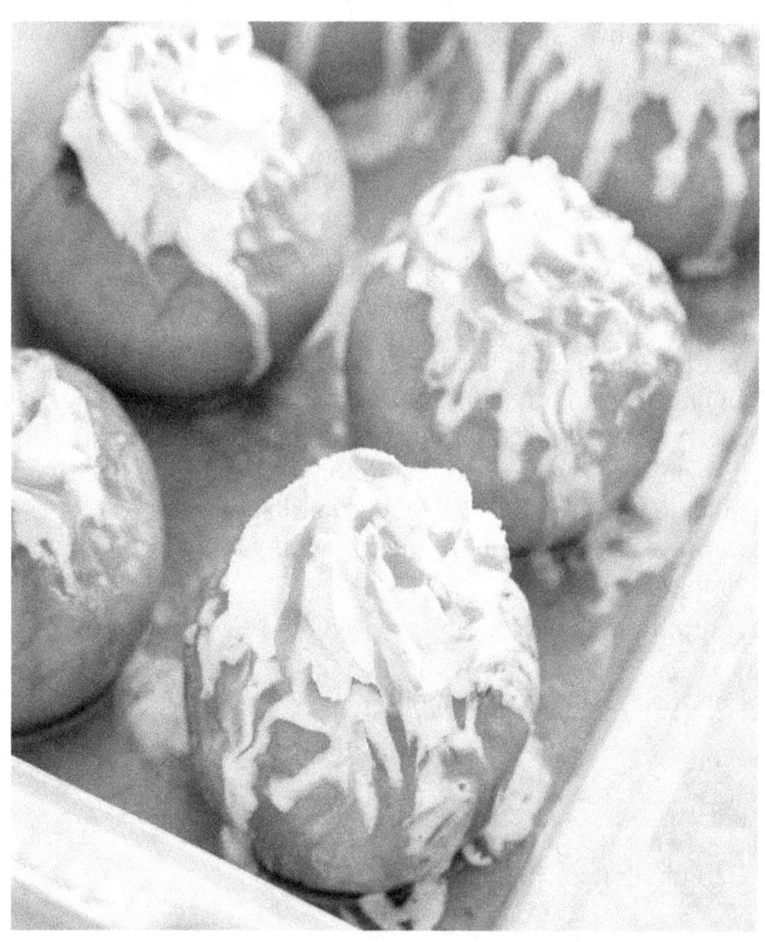

34

14.Quinoa Cake

Ingredients:

1 cup cooked quinoa

1/2 cup breadcrumbs

1/4 cup grated Parmesan cheese

1/4 cup chopped fresh herbs (such as parsley, cilantro, or basil)

1/4 cup finely chopped onion

1 clove garlic, minced

1 large egg

Salt and pepper to taste

Olive oil for frying

Preparation Method: In a large mixing bowl, add cooked quinoa, breadcrumbs, Parmesan cheese, chopped herbs, diced onion, minced garlic, and beaten egg. Season the mixture with salt and pepper to taste, then stir until completely incorporated. Form the mixture into tiny patties or cakes, using about 1/4 cup per each. In a medium-size pan, heat the olive oil. Once heated, add the quinoa cakes in batches and cook for 3-4 minutes on each side, or until golden brown and crispy. Remove the cooked quinoa cakes from the skillet and transfer to a dish lined with paper towels to drain any leftover oil. Serve the quinoa cakes warm, topped with fresh herbs as desired.

Nutritional Value per serving (approximately 2 cakes):
Calories: 200 kcal

Protein: 8g

Fat: 7g

Carbohydrates: 25g

Fiber: 3g

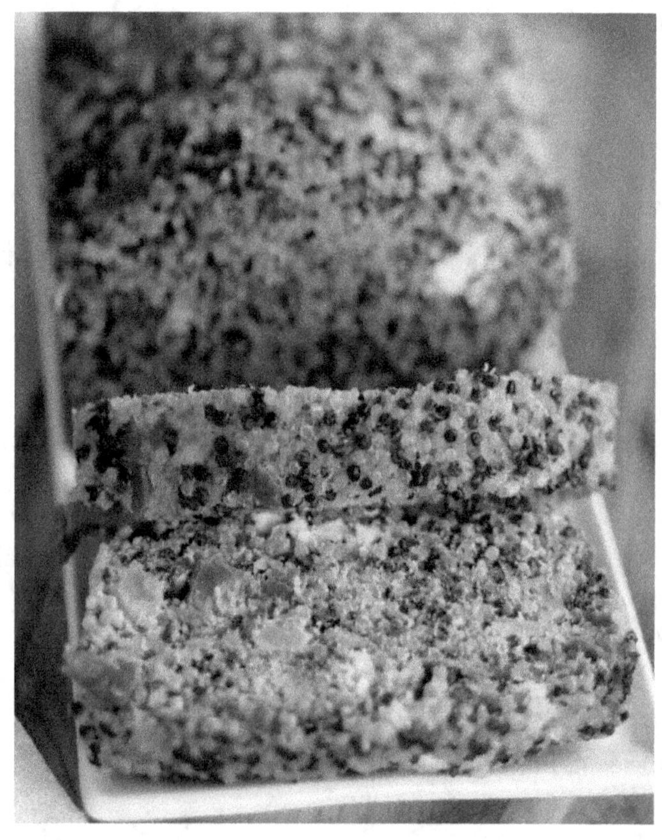

36

15. Avocado Deviled Eggs

Ingredients:

6 hard-boiled eggs

1 ripe avocado

1 tablespoon Greek yogurt

1 teaspoon Dijon mustard

1 tablespoon lemon juice

Salt and pepper to taste

Paprika for garnish

Preparation Method: Halve the hard-boiled eggs lengthwise and carefully remove the yolks. In a bowl, mash the yolks with avocado, Greek yogurt, Dijon mustard, lemon juice, salt, and pepper until smooth. Spoon the avocado mixture into the egg white halves. Sprinkle with paprika for garnish. Refrigerate until ready to serve.

Nutritional Value:

Calories: 100 kcal

Protein: 6g

Fat: 7g

Carbohydrates: 2g

Fiber: 1g

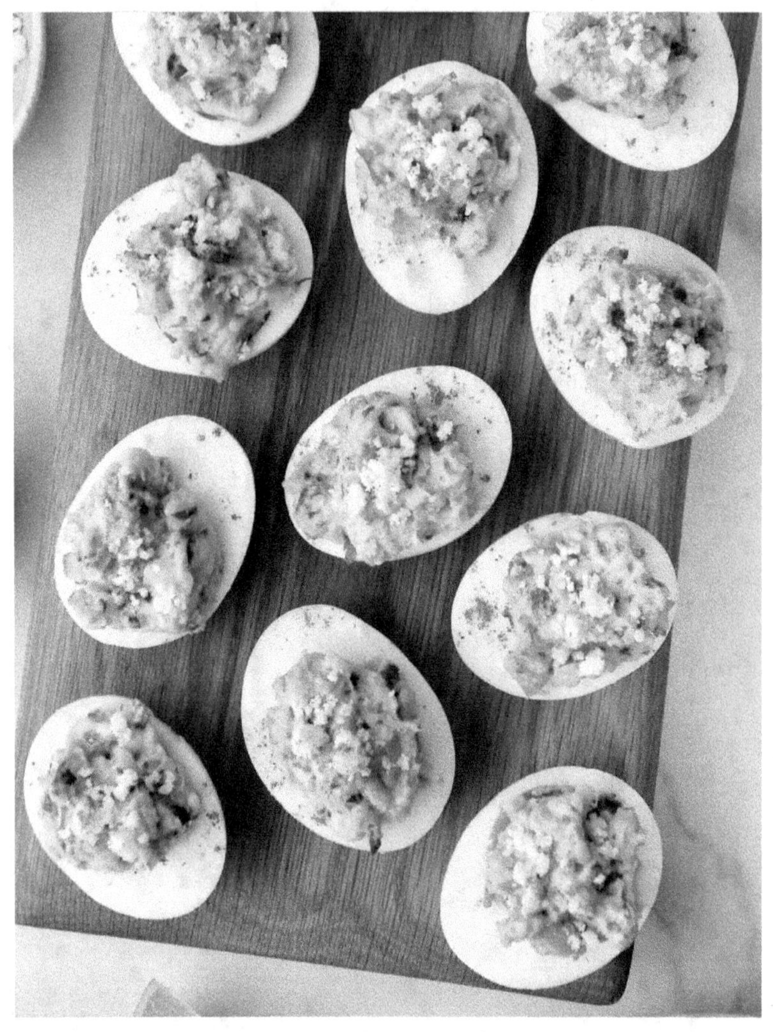

16. Baba Ghanoush

Ingredients:

2 medium eggplants

2 cloves garlic, minced

2 tablespoons tahini

2 tablespoons lemon juice

2 tablespoons olive oil

Salt and pepper to taste

Chopped parsley for garnish

Preparation Method: Preheat your grill or oven to medium-high heat. Prick the eggplants with a fork, then grill or roast until tender and browned, about 20-25 minutes. Allow the eggplants to cool, then peel and discard the skin. In a food processor, mix eggplant flesh, garlic, tahini, lemon juice, olive oil, salt, and pepper. Blend until smooth. Place the baba ghanoush in a serving basin and top with chopped parsley. Serve with pita bread or veggies to dip.

Nutritional Value:

Calories: 80 kcal

Protein: 2g

Fat: 7g

Carbohydrates: 5g

Fiber: 3g

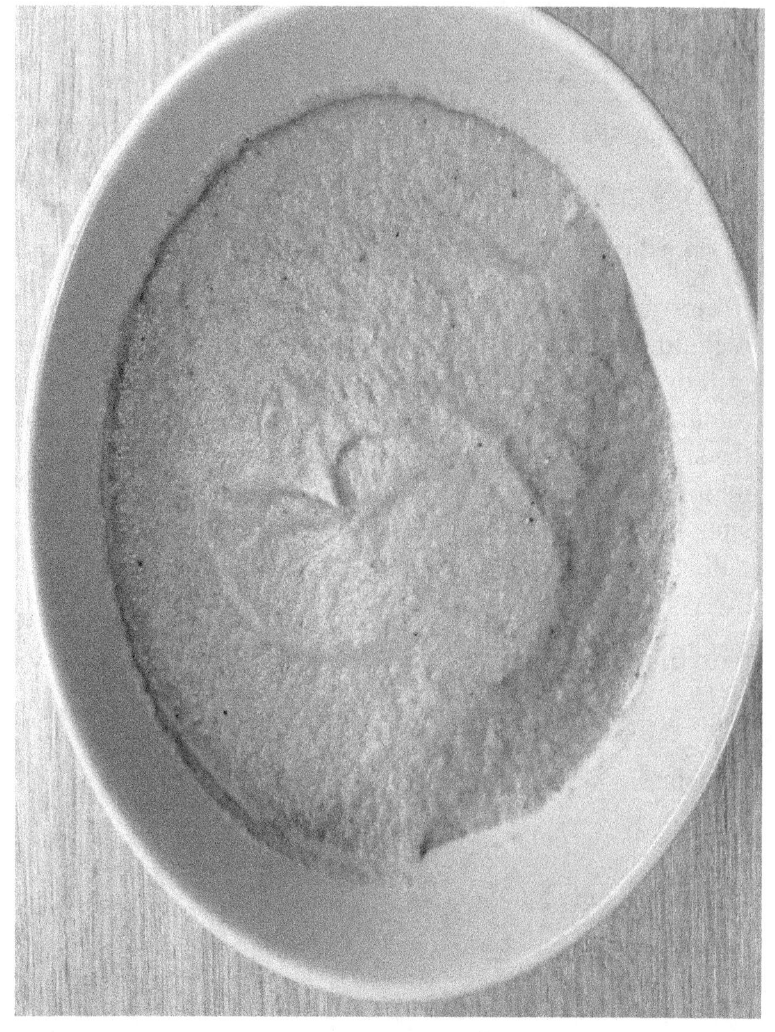

17. Fruit Salsa and Sweet Chips

Ingredients:

2 apples, diced

1 cup strawberries, diced

1 kiwi, diced

1 tablespoon honey

Juice of 1 lime

Cinnamon sugar tortilla chips

Preparation Method: In a bowl, combine the diced apples, strawberries, and kiwi. Drizzle with honey and lime juice, and toss gently to combine. Refrigerate for at least 30 minutes to allow the flavors to meld. Serve the fruit salsa with cinnamon sugar tortilla chips for dipping.

Nutritional Values:

Calories: 120 kcal

Protein: 1g

Fat: 0g

Carbohydrates: 30g

Fiber: 3g

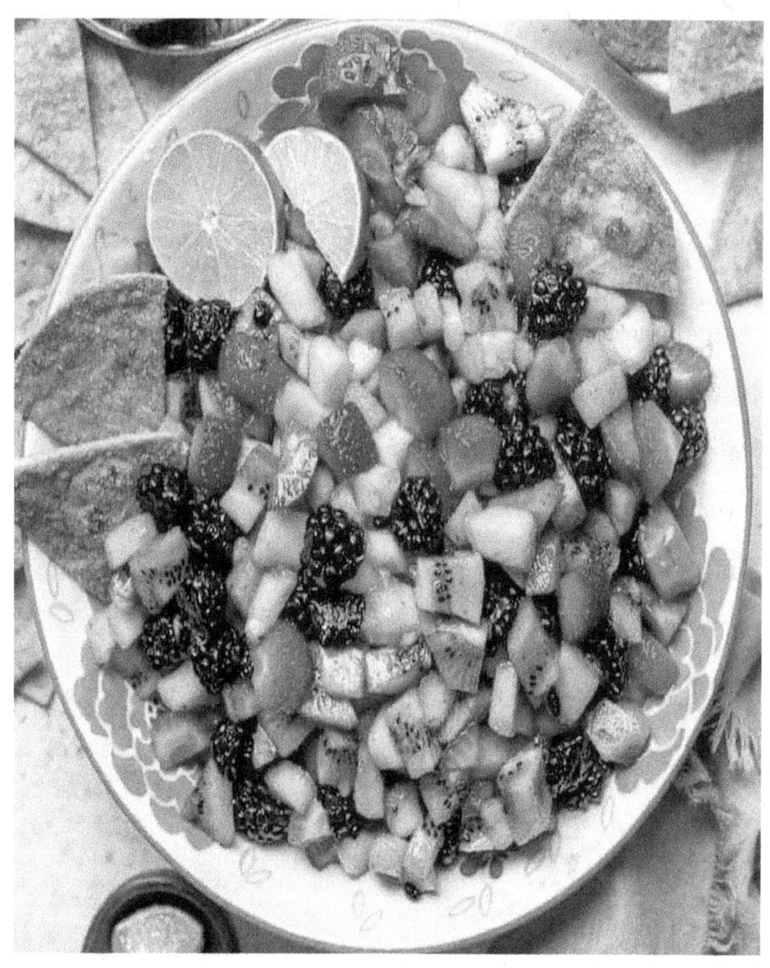

18. Grilled Pineapple

Ingredients:

1 pineapple, peeled, cored, and cut into rings

Honey or brown sugar (optional)

Cinnamon (optional)

Preparation Method: Preheat grill to medium-high heat. Grill pineapple rings for 2-3 minutes on each side, or until grill marks appear. Optionally, brush with honey or sprinkle with brown sugar and cinnamon for added sweetness. Serve grilled pineapple as a side dish or dessert.

Nutritional Values:

Calories: 80 kcal

Protein: 1g

Fat: 0g

Carbohydrates: 20g

Fiber: 2g

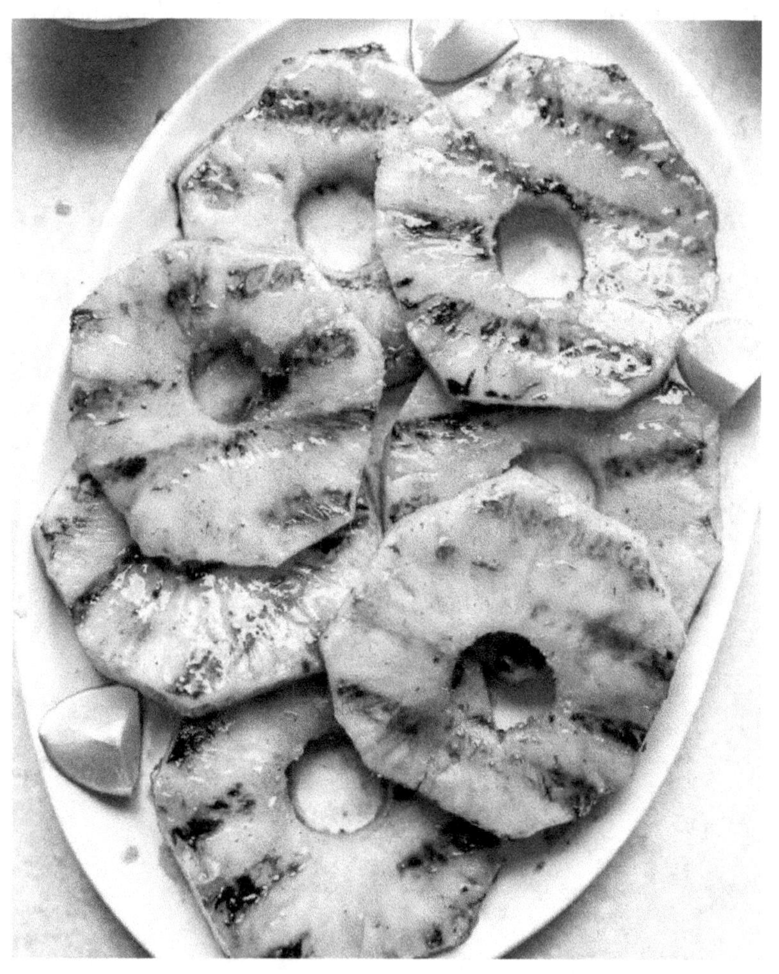

19. Hummus

Ingredients:

1 can (15 oz) chickpeas, drained and rinsed

2 cloves garlic

2 tablespoons tahini

2 tablespoons lemon juice

2 tablespoons olive oil

Salt and pepper to taste

Water (as needed for consistency)

Preparation Method: In a food processor, mix the chickpeas, garlic, tahini, lemon juice, olive oil, salt, and pepper. Blend until smooth, adding water as required to get desired consistency. Season to taste. Transfer the hummus to a serving bowl, drizzle with olive oil, and top with paprika to garnish. Serve with pita bread or veggies to dip.

Nutritional Values:

Calories: 70 kcal

Protein: 3g

Fat: 5g

Carbohydrates: 4g

Fiber: 2g

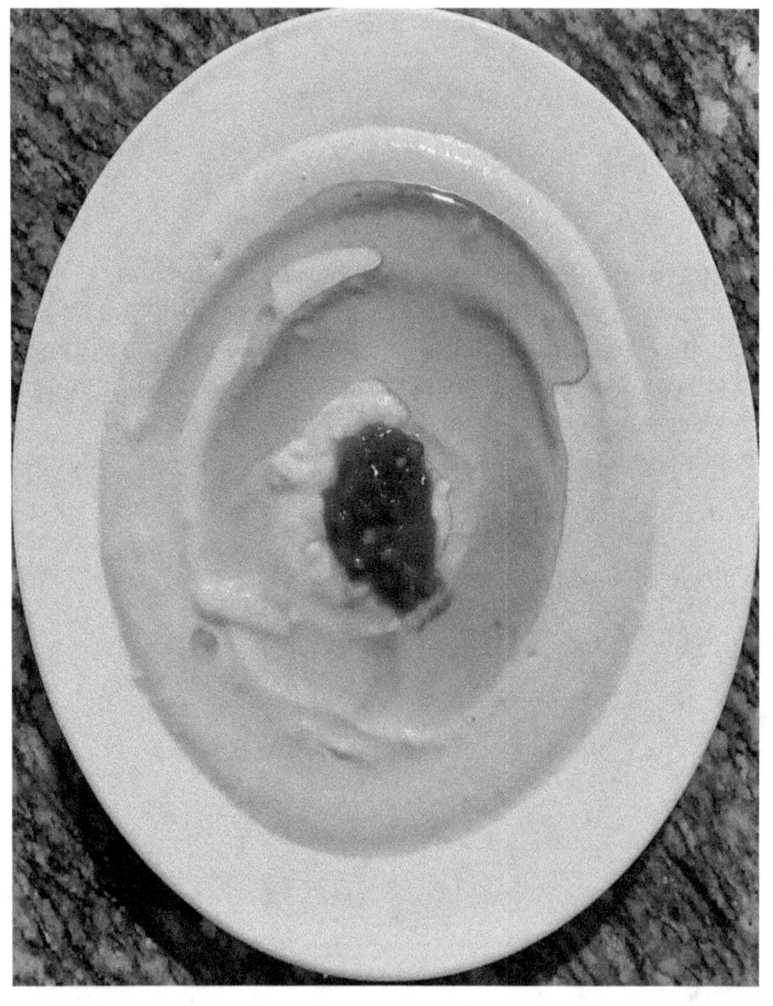

20. Peanut Butter Hummus

Ingredients:

1 can (15 oz) chickpeas, drained and rinsed

1/4 cup peanut butter

2 tablespoons maple syrup or honey

2 tablespoons lemon juice

2 tablespoons olive oil

1/4 teaspoon ground cinnamon (optional)

Water (as needed for consistency)

Salt to taste

Preparation Method: In a food processor, combine chickpeas, peanut butter, maple syrup or honey, lemon juice, olive oil, and ground cinnamon. Blend until smooth, adding water as needed for desired consistency. Adjust seasoning to taste with salt. Transfer peanut butter hummus to a serving bowl. Serve with fruit, crackers, or vegetables for dipping.

Nutritional Values:

Calories: 90 kcal

Protein: 4g

Fat: 6g

Carbohydrates: 5g

Fiber: 2g

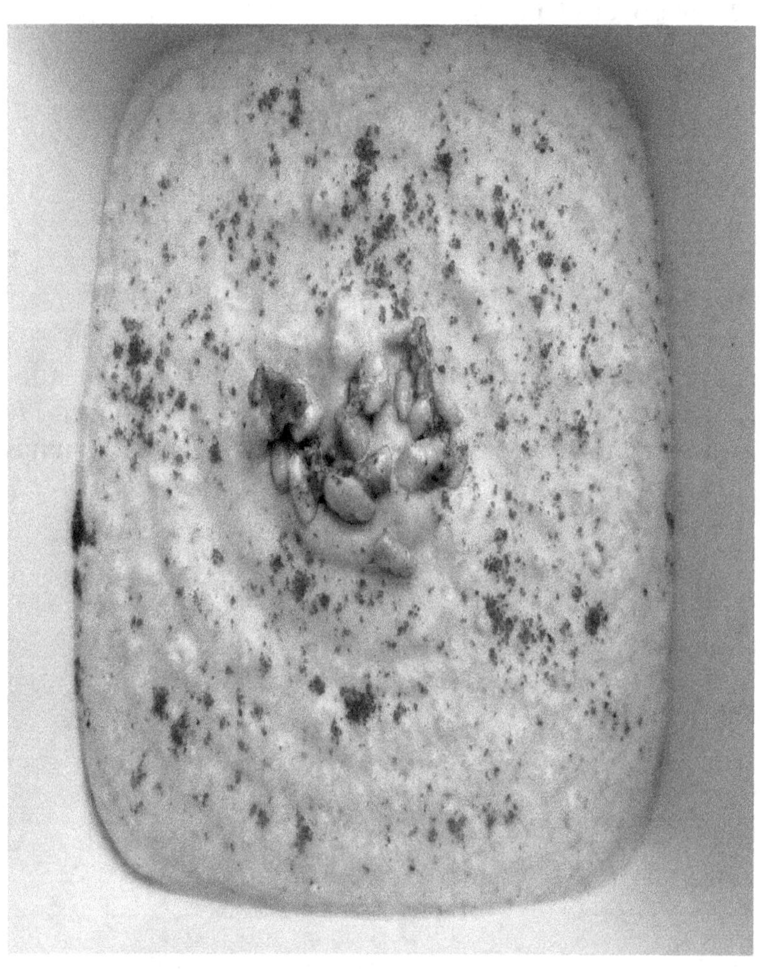

48

21. Pickled Asparagus

Ingredients:

1 bunch asparagus, trimmed

1 cup white vinegar

1 cup water

2 tablespoons sugar

1 tablespoon salt

2 cloves garlic, smashed

1 teaspoon black peppercorns

1 teaspoon mustard seeds

Preparation: Blanch the asparagus in boiling water for 1-2 minutes before transferring to an ice bath to halt the cooking process. In a saucepan, mix together white vinegar, water, sugar, salt, garlic, black peppercorns, and mustard seeds. Bring to a boil, then decrease heat and let simmer for 5 minutes. Pack the blanched asparagus into sterilized jars and pour the hot brine over them. Seal and cool jars before refrigerating for 24hrs.

Nutritional Values:

Calories: 10 kcal

Protein: 1g

Fat: 0g

Carbohydrates: 2g

Fiber: 1g

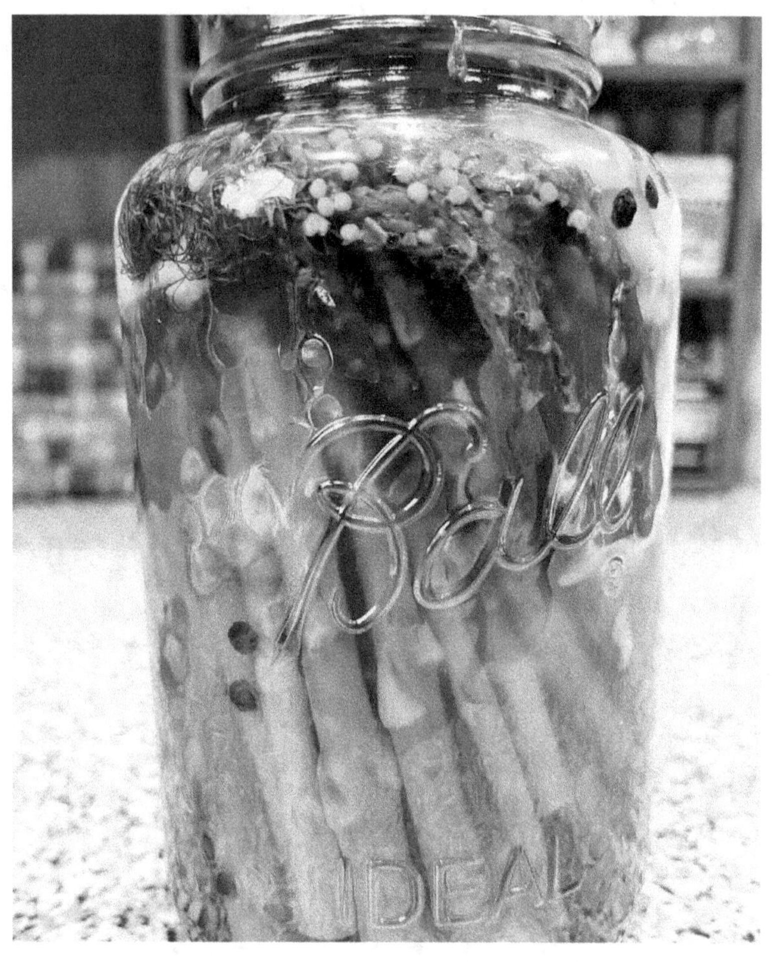
Ball
IDEAL

22. 6-Grain Hot Cereal

Ingredients:

1/4 cup 6-grain hot cereal mix

1 cup water or milk

Optional toppings: fruits, nuts, honey, cinnamon

Preparation Method: In a saucepan, bring water or milk to a boil. Stir in the 6-grain hot cereal mix. Reduce heat to low and simmer for about 5 minutes, stirring occasionally, until thickened. Serve hot with your choice of toppings.

Nutritional Value per serving:

Calories: 150 kcal

Protein: 5g

Fat: 2g

Carbohydrates: 30g

Fiber: 5g

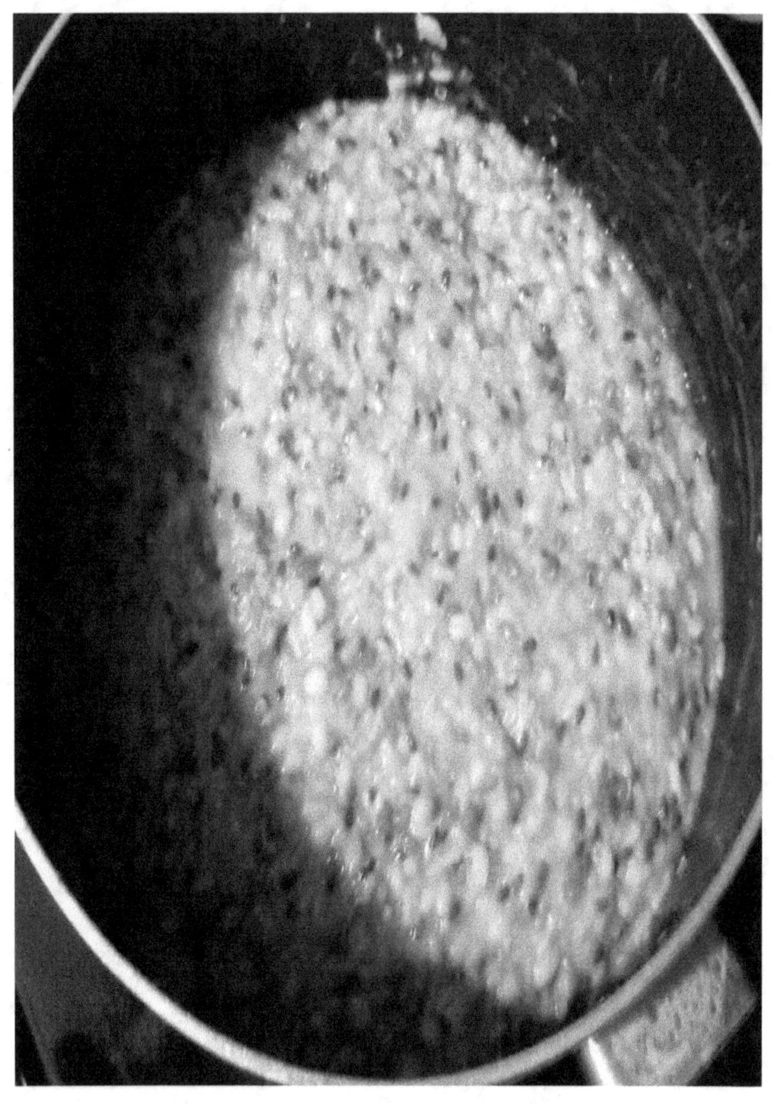

23. Beef and Vegetable Kebabs

Ingredients:

Cubed beef

Assorted vegetables (such as bell peppers, onions, zucchini)

Marinade ingredients (your choice)

Skewers

Preparation Method: Marinate cubed beef in your choice of marinade for at least 30 minutes. Thread marinated beef and assorted vegetables onto skewers. Grill or broil kebabs until beef is cooked to desired doneness and vegetables are tender.

Nutritional Value Per Serving:

Calories: 250-350 kcal

Protein: 20-30g

Fat: 10-15g

Carbohydrates: 10-15g

Fiber: 2-4g

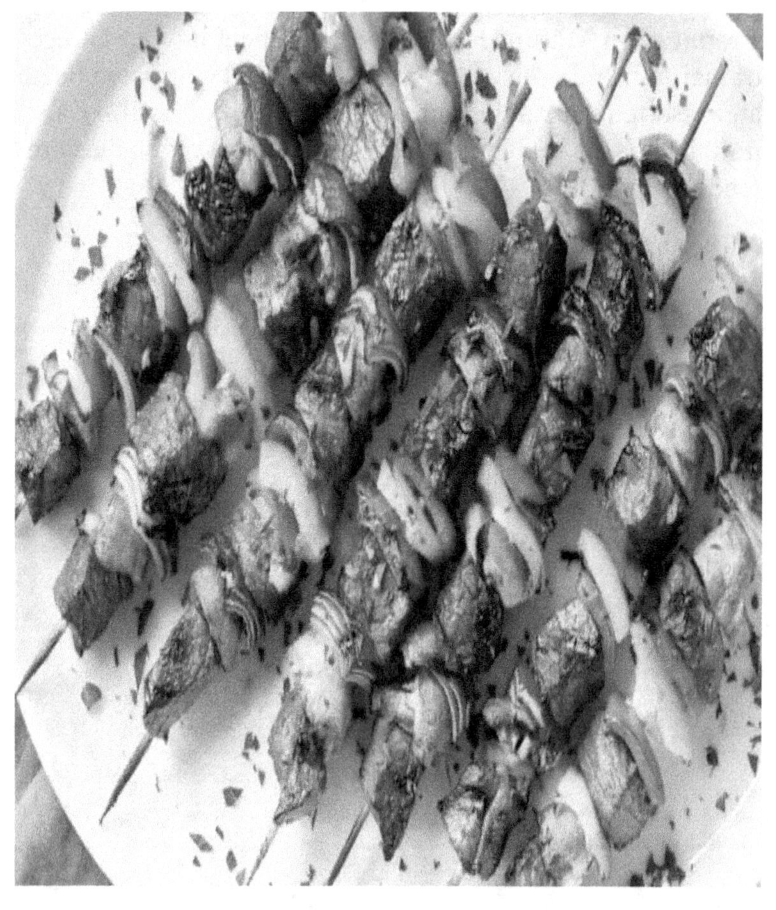

24. Broccoli Garlic and Rigatoni

Ingredients:

Rigatoni pasta

Broccoli florets

Garlic cloves, minced

Olive oil

Parmesan cheese

Salt and pepper

Preparation Method: Rigatoni pasta should be cooked as directed on the package. Drain and set aside. In a skillet, cook the minced garlic in olive oil until aromatic. Add the broccoli florets and simmer until tender. Toss cooked spaghetti with the broccoli and garlic combination. Season with salt and pepper, then top with Parmesan cheese before serving.

Nutritional Value Per Serving:

Calories: 300-400 kcal

Protein: 10-15g

Fat: 5-10g

Carbohydrates: 50-60g

Fiber: 5-8g

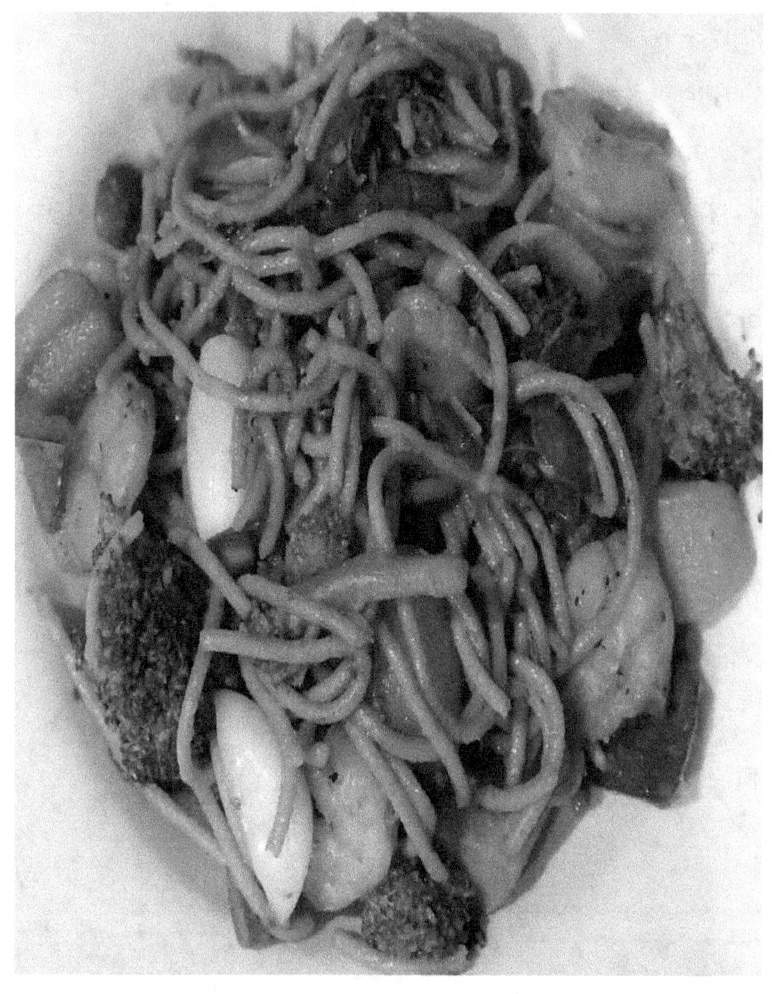

25. Chicken Brats

Ingredients:

Chicken bratwurst sausages

Whole wheat buns

Assorted toppings (such as sauerkraut, mustard, onions)

Preparation Method: Grill or pan-fry the chicken brats until well done. Serve on whole wheat buns with your choice of toppings.

Nutritional Value Per Serving:

Calories: 150-250 kcal

Protein: 15-20g

Fat: 8-12g

Carbohydrates: 0-5g

Fiber: 0-1g

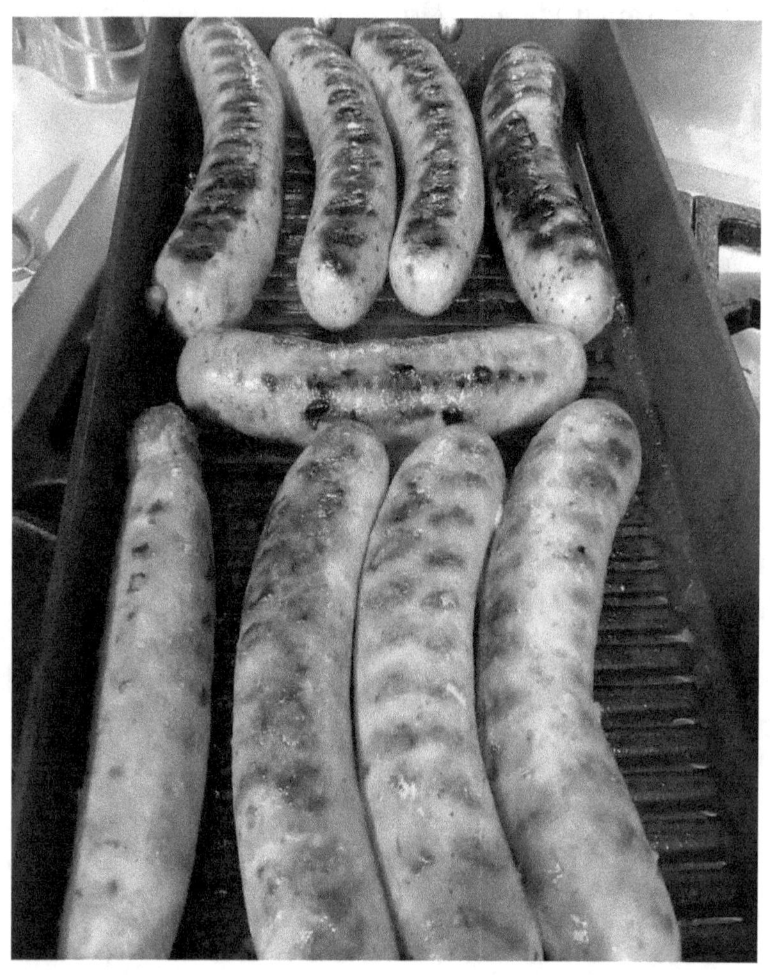

26. Chicken Salad with Pineapple and Balsamic Vinaigrette

Ingredients:

Cooked chicken breast, diced

Mixed salad greens

Pineapple chunks

Cherry tomatoes

Cucumber slices

Balsamic vinaigrette dressing

Preparation Method: In a large bowl, combine diced chicken breast, mixed salad greens, pineapple chunks, cherry tomatoes, and cucumber slices. Drizzle with balsamic vinaigrette dressing and toss to coat evenly. Serve immediately.

Nutritional Value Per Serving:

Calories: 250-350 kcal

Protein: 20-25g

Fat: 10-15g

Carbohydrates: 15-20g

Fiber: 3-5g

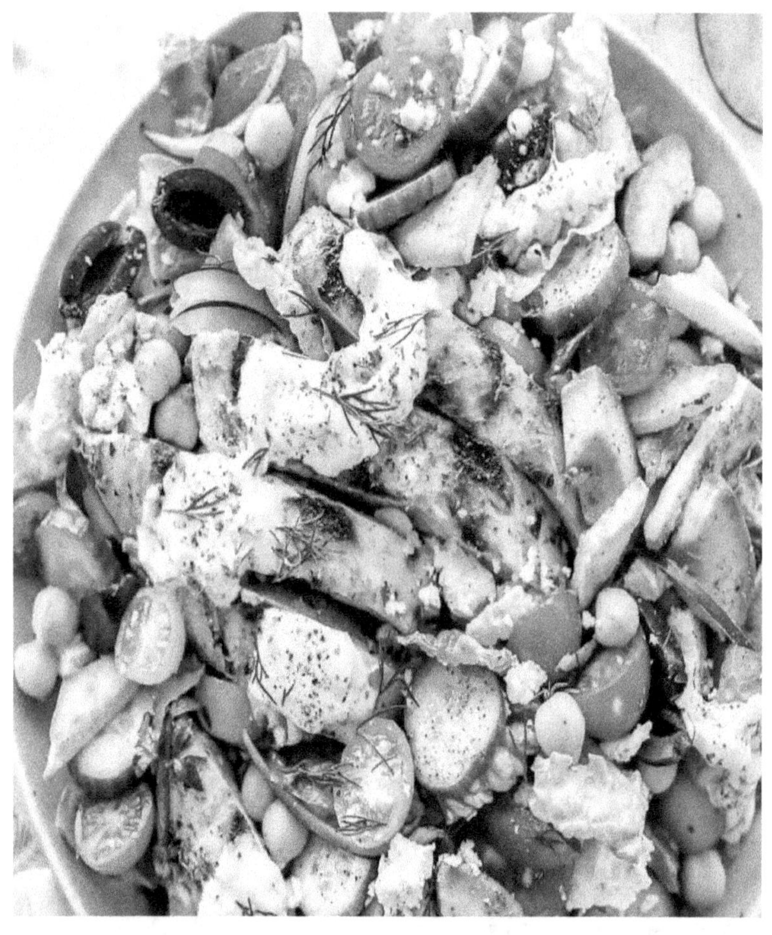

27. Corn Tamales with Avocado-Tomatillo Salsa

Ingredients for Corn Tamales:

2 cups masa harina (corn flour)

1 cup vegetable broth

1 cup corn kernels

1/4 cup melted butter or vegetable oil

1 teaspoon baking powder

Salt to taste

Corn husks, soaked in warm water for 30 minutes

Ingredients for Avocado-Tomatillo Salsa:

2 ripe avocados, diced

4 tomatillos, husked and diced

1/4 cup chopped cilantro

1 jalapeño, seeded and minced

Juice of 1 lime

Preparation for Corn Tamales: In a mixing bowl, combine masa harina, vegetable broth, melted butter or oil, baking powder, salt, and corn kernels. Mix until a soft dough forms. Spread a thin layer of the masa mixture onto each soaked corn husk. Place a spoonful of filling in the center of the masa. Roll up the corn husk to enclose the filling and tie with kitchen twine. Steam tamales for about 45-60 minutes, or until the masa is firm.

Preparation for Avocado-Tomatillo Salsa: In a bowl, combine diced avocados, tomatillos, cilantro, jalapeño, lime juice, and salt. Mix gently until well combined.

Nutritional Value Per Serving:

Calories: 250 kcal

Protein: 5g

Fat: 12g

Carbohydrates: 30g

Fiber: 5g

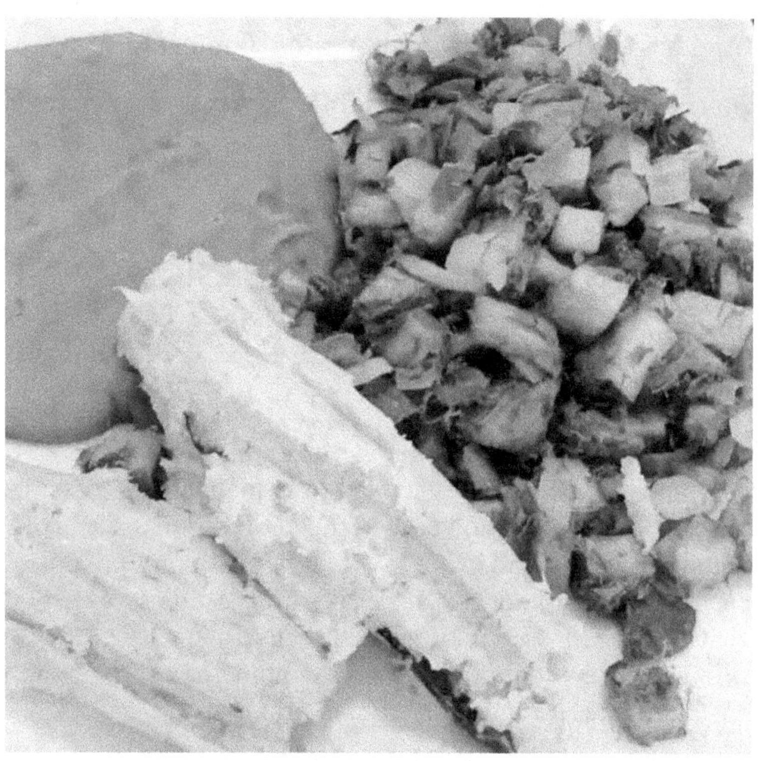

28. Fish Tacos with Tomatillo Sauce

Ingredients for Fish Tacos:

1 lb white fish fillets (such as cod or tilapia)

8 small corn tortillas

1 cup shredded cabbage

1 avocado, sliced

Lime wedges, for serving

Fresh cilantro, for garnish

Ingredients for Tomatillo Sauce:

4 tomatillos, husked and quartered

1/2 onion, chopped

2 cloves garlic, minced

1 jalapeño, seeded and chopped

1/4 cup chopped cilantro

Juice of 1 lime

Salt to taste

Preparation Method for Fish Tacos: Season fish fillets with salt and pepper. Grill or pan-sear the fish until it is cooked through. Warm the corn tortillas on a griddle or pan. Make tacos using cooked fish, shredded cabbage, sliced avocado, and tomatillo salsa. Serve with lime wedges and a garnish of fresh cilantro.

Preparation for Tomatillo Sauce: whisk together quartered tomatillos, chopped onion, minced garlic, diced jalapeño, cilantro, lime juice, and salt. Blend until smooth.

Nutritional Value Per Serving:

Calories: 200-300 kcal

Protein: 15-25g

Fat: 5-10g

Carbohydrates: 20-30g

Fiber: 3-5g

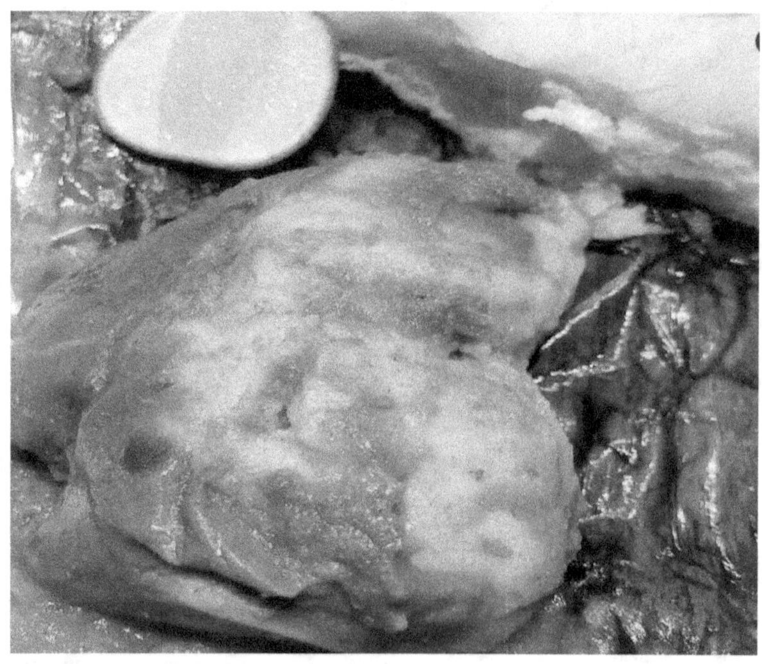

29. Mango Salsa Pizza

Ingredients for Mango Salsa:

1 ripe mango, diced

1/2 red onion, finely chopped

1 red bell pepper, diced

1 jalapeño, seeded and minced

Juice of 1 lime

2 tablespoons chopped cilantro

Salt to taste

Ingredients for Pizza:

Prepared pizza dough

Olive oil

Mozzarella cheese, shredded

Cooked chicken breast, diced

Mango salsa (from above)

Preparation Method for Mango Salsa: In a bowl, mix diced mango, red onion, red bell pepper, minced jalapeño, lime juice, cilantro, and salt. Combine thoroughly and chill until ready to use.

Preparation Method for Pizza: Preheat the oven to the proper temperature for your pizza dough. Roll the pizza dough out to the appropriate thickness on a lightly floured board. Move the dough to a pizza stone or baking sheet.

Brush the dough with olive oil and cover with shredded mozzarella cheese. Top with diced cooked chicken breasts and a large serving of mango salsa. Bake in the preheated oven until the crust is golden brown and the cheese has melted and bubbled. Remove from the oven, cut into slices, and serve hot.

Nutritional Value Per Serving:

Calories: 250-350 kcal

Protein: 8-12g

Fat: 8-12g

Carbohydrates: 30-40g

Fiber: 3-5g

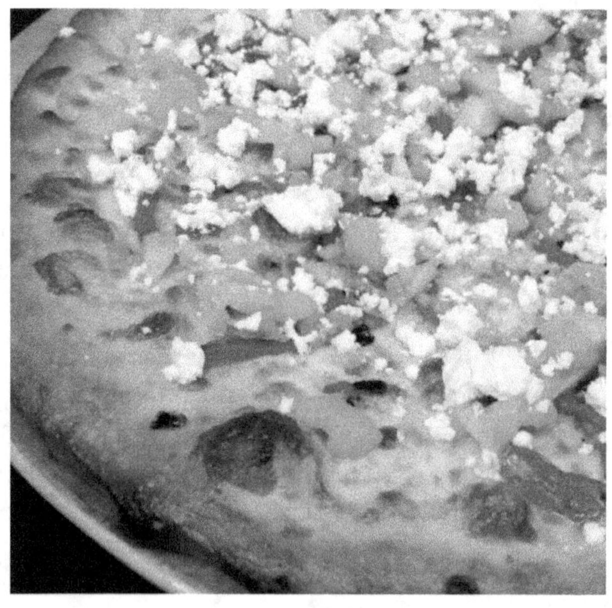

30. Grilled Pork Fajitas

Ingredients:

Pork tenderloin, sliced into strips

Bell peppers, sliced

Onion, sliced

Fajita seasoning

Flour tortillas

Toppings: sour cream, guacamole, salsa, shredded cheese

Preparation Method: Season the pork strips with fajita spice. Place a grill or grill pan over medium-high heat. Grill the pork strips, bell peppers, and onions until they are well cooked and slightly browned. Warm flour tortillas on the grill. Prepare fajitas using grilled pork, bell peppers, and onions. Serve with your choice of toppings.

Nutritional Value Per Serving:

Calories: 300-400 kcal

Protein: 20-25g

Fat: 10-15g

Carbohydrates: 20-30g

Fiber: 3-5g

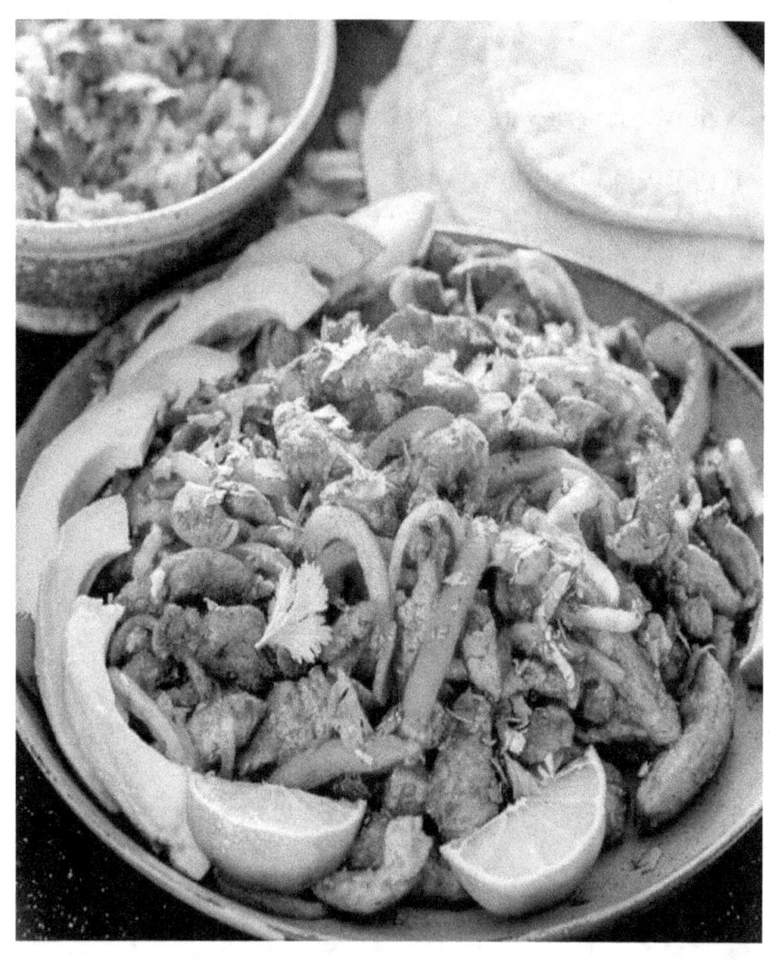

31. Rice Noodles with Spring Vegetables

Ingredients:

Rice noodles

Assorted spring vegetables (such as snap peas, asparagus, carrots)

Garlic, minced

Soy sauce

Sesame oil

Sesame seeds for garnish

Optional protein: tofu, shrimp, or chicken

Preparation Method: Cook rice noodles according to package instructions. Drain and set aside. In a pan, sauté minced garlic in sesame oil until fragrant. Add assorted spring vegetables and cook until tender-crisp. Toss cooked rice noodles with the sautéed vegetables and soy sauce. Serve hot, garnished with sesame seeds.

Nutritional Value Per Serving:

Calories: 250-350 kcal

Protein: 5-10g

Fat: 5-10g

Carbohydrates: 40-50g

Fiber: 5-8g

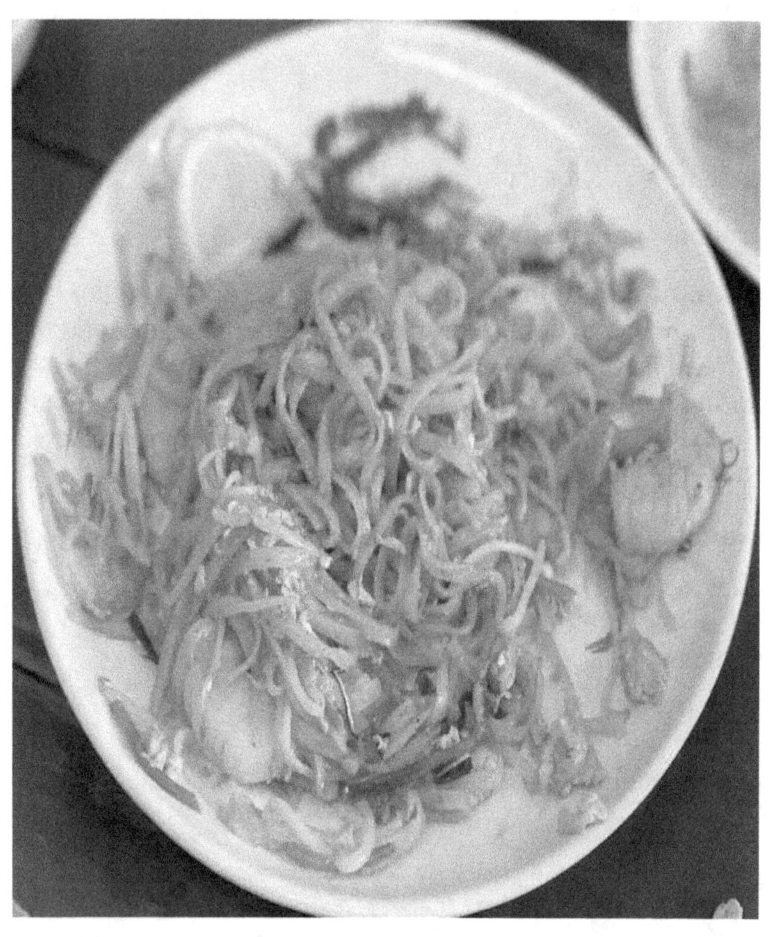

32. Smoky Bean and Mushroom Cornucopias

Ingredients:

Puff pastry sheets

Canned black beans, drained and rinsed

Mushrooms, sliced

Onion, diced

Garlic, minced

Smoked paprika

Cumin

Salt and pepper

Olive oil

Preparation Method: Preheat the oven to the temperature recommended for the puff pastry. Heat olive oil in a skillet over medium heat. Sauté diced onion and minced garlic until softened. Add sliced mushrooms and cook until they release their moisture and become tender. Stir in drained black beans, smoked paprika, cumin, salt, and pepper. Cook for a few more minutes until heated through. Roll out the puff pastry sheets and cut them into squares or rectangles. Place a spoonful of the bean and mushroom mixture onto each puff pastry square. Fold the pastry over the filling to form a triangle shape, pinching the edges to seal. Bake in the preheated oven until the puff pastry is golden brown and crispy. Serve hot as an appetizer or snack.

Nutritional Value Per Serving:

Calories: 200-300 kcal

Protein: 8-12g

Fat: 5-8g

Carbohydrates: 30-40g

Fiber: 5-8g

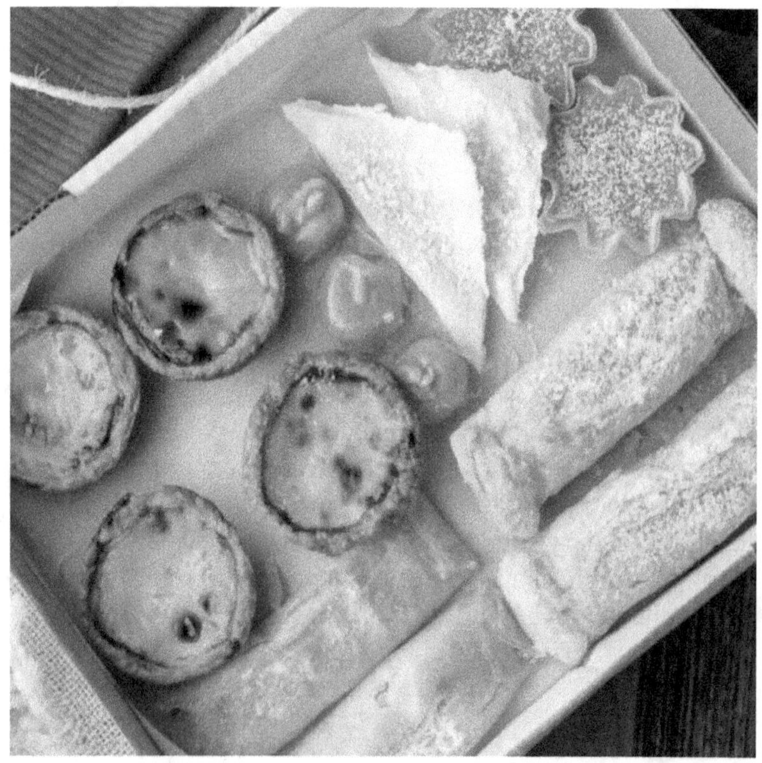

33. Whole-Wheat Blueberry Pancakes

Ingredients:

Whole-wheat flour

Baking powder

Salt

Milk (dairy or plant-based)

Eggs

Vanilla extract

Fresh blueberries

Preparation Method: In a large mixing bowl, whisk together whole-wheat flour, baking powder, and salt. In a separate bowl, whisk together milk, eggs, and vanilla extract. Pour the wet ingredients into the dry ingredients and stir until just combined. Do not overmix. Gently fold in fresh blueberries. Heat a lightly greased skillet or griddle over medium heat. Pour about 1/4 cup of batter onto the skillet for each pancake. Cook until bubbles form on the surface of the pancake, then flip and cook until golden brown on both sides. Serve warm with maple syrup and additional blueberries if desired.

Nutritional Value Per Serving:

Calories: 150-250 kcal

Protein: 5-8g

Fat: 3-5g

Carbohydrates: 20-30g

Fiber: 3-5g

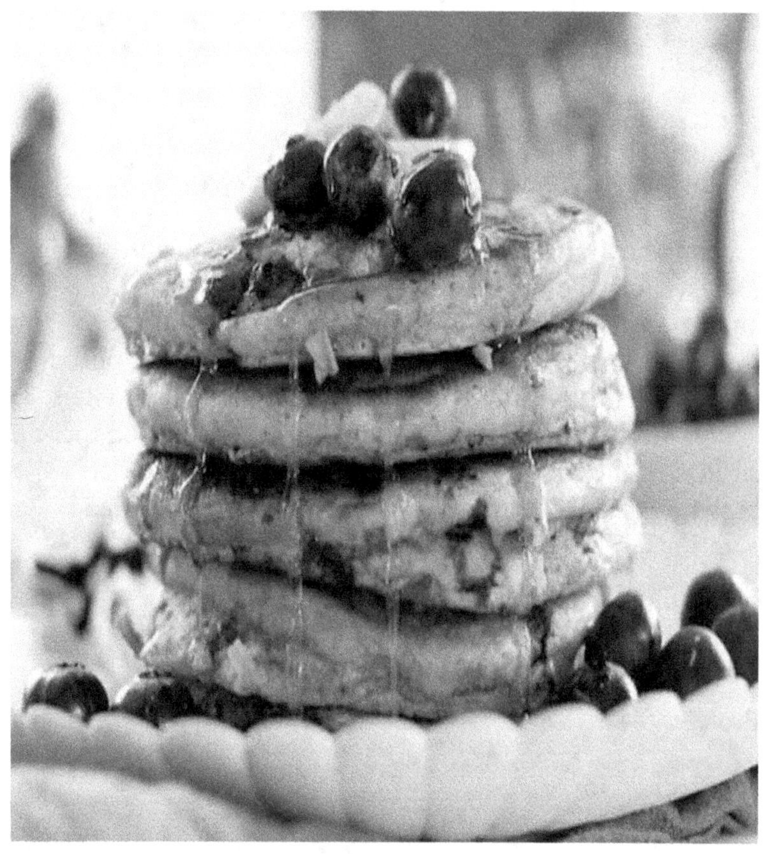

34. Caramelized Balsamic Vinaigrette

Ingredients:

1/2 cup balsamic vinegar

2 tablespoons honey or maple syrup

1 clove garlic, minced

1/2 cup olive oil

Salt and pepper to taste

Preparation Method: In a small saucepan, heat the balsamic vinegar and honey over medium heat. Stir in the minced garlic and continue cooking until the mixture is reduced by half and becomes syrupy, about 10-15 minutes. Remove from heat and let cool slightly. Gradually whisk in the olive oil until emulsified. Season with salt and pepper to taste. Store in a sealed container in the refrigerator for up to a week.

Approximate Nutritional Value (per serving):

Calories: 120 kcal

Protein: 0g

Fat: 14g

Carbohydrates: 6g

Fiber: 0g

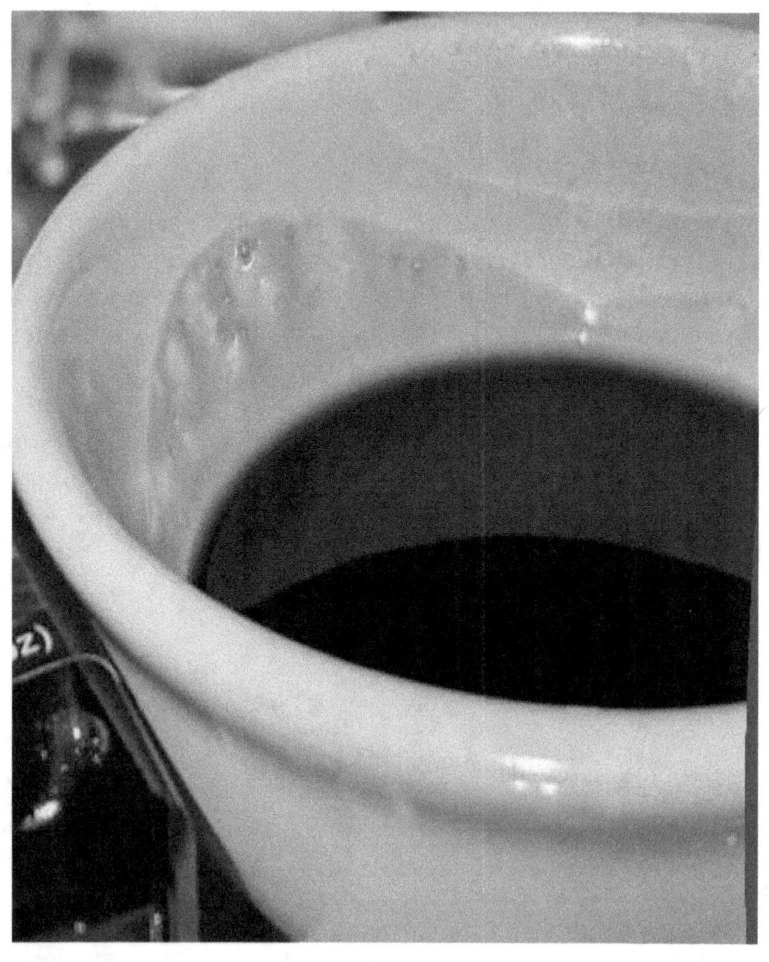

35. House Ranch Dressing

Ingredients:

1 cup mayonnaise

1/2 cup sour cream

1/4 cup buttermilk

2 tablespoons chopped fresh parsley

1 tablespoon chopped fresh dill

1 clove garlic, minced

1 teaspoon onion powder

1 teaspoon dried chives

Salt and pepper to taste

Preparation Method: In a mixing bowl, whisk together mayonnaise, sour cream, and buttermilk until smooth. Stir in chopped parsley, dill, minced garlic, onion powder, and dried chives. Season with salt and pepper to taste. Refrigerate for at least 1 hour before serving to allow flavors to meld.

Approximate Nutritional Value (per serving):

Calories: 160 kcal

Protein: 1g

Fat: 17g

Carbohydrates: 2g

Fiber: 0g

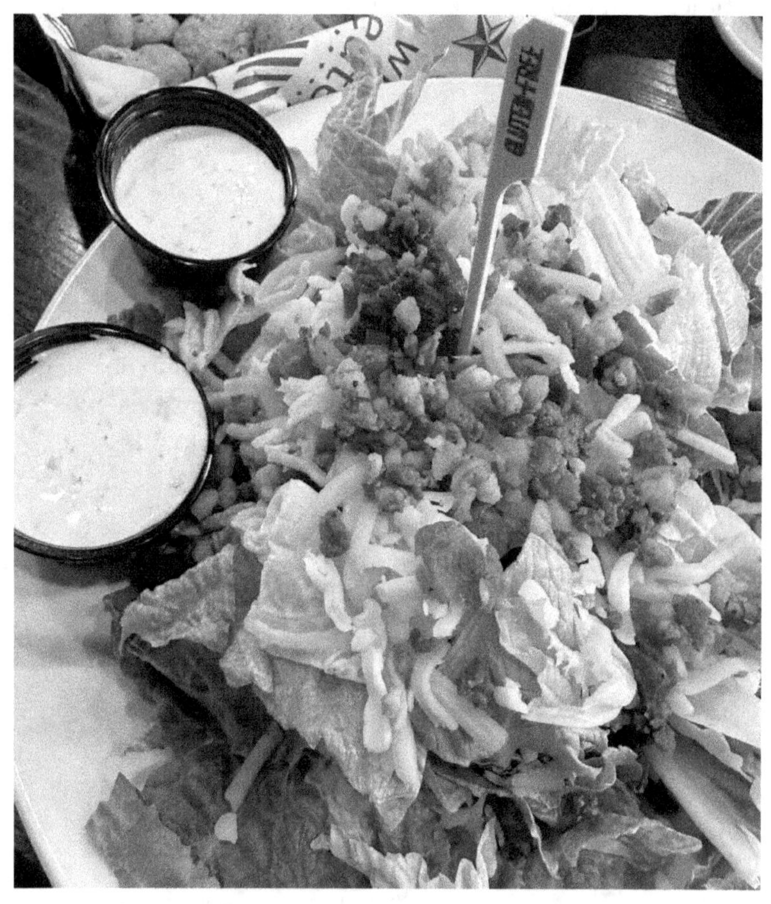

GLUTEN FREE

36. Peach Honey Spread

Ingredients:

2 ripe peaches, peeled and diced

2 tablespoons honey

1 tablespoon lemon juice

Preparation Method: Dice the peaches and purée them in a blender or food processor until smooth. Transfer the puree to a small saucepan and mix in the honey and lemon juice. Cook over low heat, stirring periodically, for 15-20 minutes, or until the mixture thickens to a spreadable consistency. Allow it cool fully before transferring to a jar or container.

Approximate Nutritional Value (per serving):

Calories: 45 kcal

Protein: 0g

Fat: 0g

Carbohydrates: 12g

Fiber: 1g

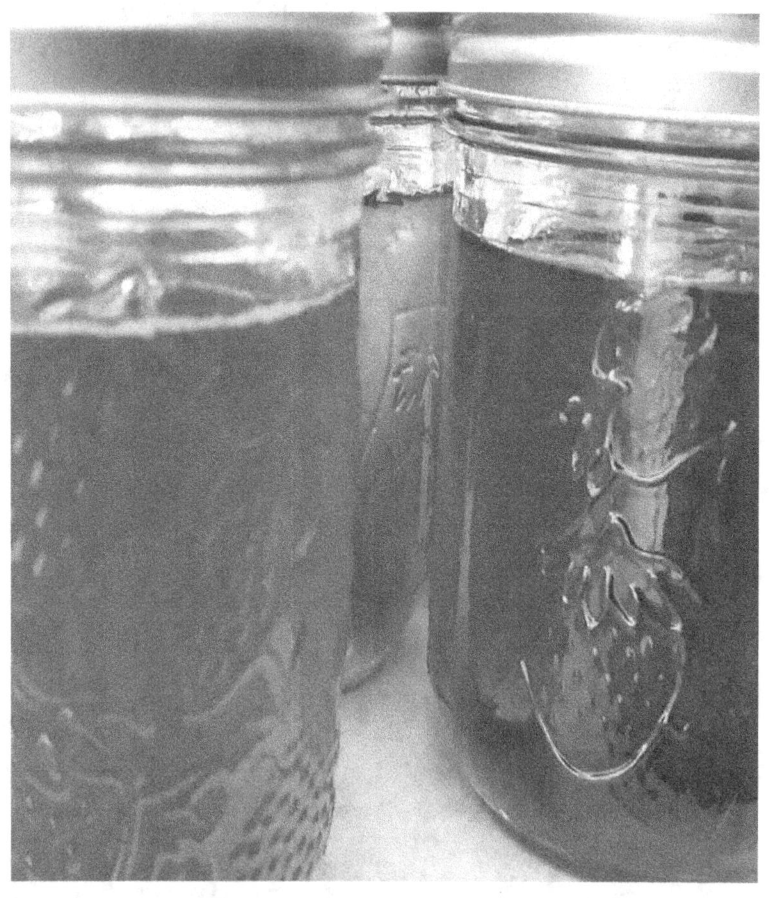

37. Roasted Bell Pepper Pineapple Salsa

Ingredients:

1 red bell pepper

1 cup diced pineapple

1/4 cup finely chopped red onion

1 jalapeño, seeded and minced

2 tablespoons chopped fresh cilantro

Juice of 1 lime

Salt and pepper to taste

Preparation Method: Preheat broiler to high. Place the whole red bell pepper on a baking sheet and broil, turning occasionally, until charred and blistered on all sides, about 10-15 minutes. Remove the bell pepper from the oven and transfer to a bowl. Allow it to steam for 10 minutes while covered with plastic wrap. Peel off the charred skin, remove the seeds and stem, and dice the roasted bell pepper. In a mixing bowl, combine diced roasted bell pepper, diced pineapple, chopped red onion, minced jalapeño, chopped cilantro, and lime juice. Season with salt and pepper to taste. Refrigerate for at least 30 minutes before serving to enable flavors to blend.

Approximate Nutritional Value (per serving):

Calories: 30 kcal

Protein: 0g

Fat: 0g

Carbohydrates: 8g

Fiber: 1g

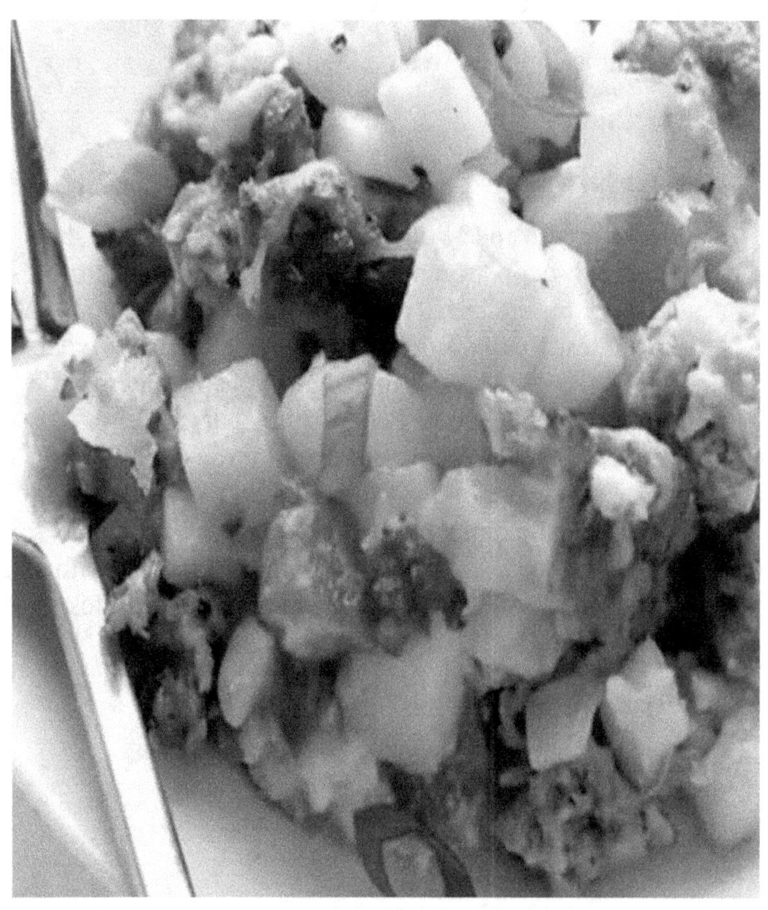

38. Yellow Pear and Cherry Tomato Salad

Ingredients:

2 cups yellow pear tomatoes, halved

1 cup cherry tomatoes, halved

1/4 cup red onion, thinly sliced

2 tablespoons fresh basil, chopped

1 tablespoon extra-virgin olive oil

1 tablespoon balsamic vinegar

Salt and pepper to taste

Preparation Method: In a large bowl, combine the yellow pear tomatoes, cherry tomatoes, red onion, and fresh basil. Drizzle with olive oil and balsamic vinegar. Season with salt and pepper. Toss gently to coat evenly. Allow the salad to settle for approximately 10 minutes so that the flavors may blend.

Approximate Nutritional Value (per serving):

Calories: 60 kcal

Protein: 1g

Fat: 4g

Carbohydrates: 6g

Fiber: 2g

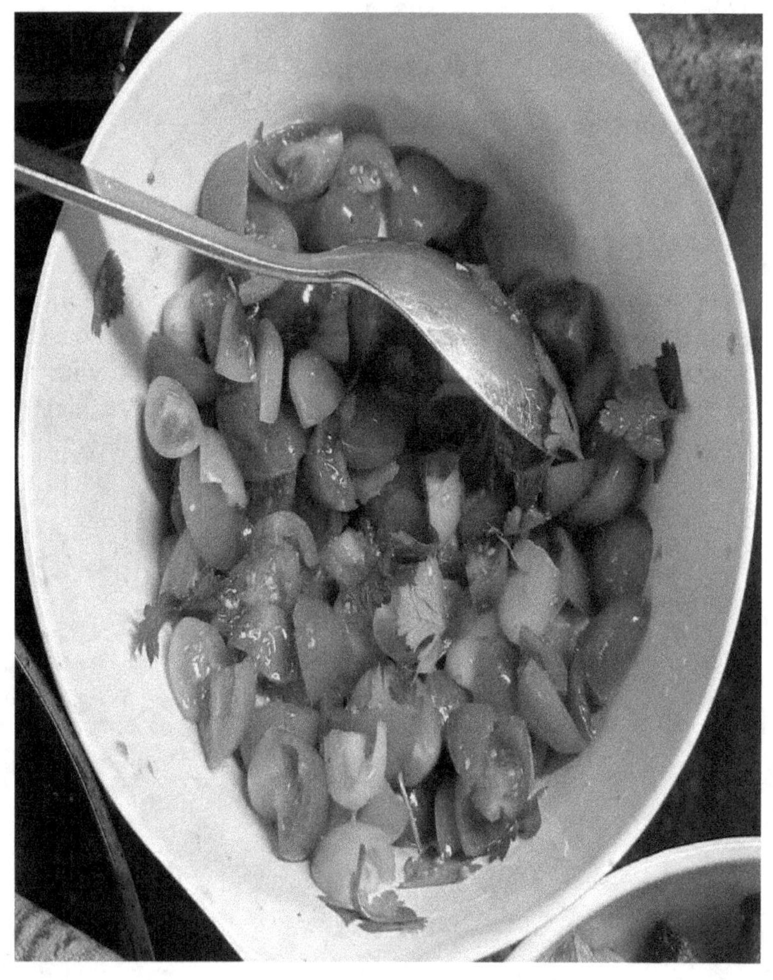

39. Warm Coleslaw with Honey Dressing

Ingredients:

4 cups shredded green cabbage

1 cup shredded carrots

1/4 cup apple cider vinegar

2 tablespoons honey

1 tablespoon Dijon mustard

2 tablespoons olive oil

Salt and pepper to taste

Preparation Method: In a large skillet, heat olive oil over medium heat. Add shredded cabbage and carrots to the skillet and cook until slightly wilted, about 5-7 minutes. In a small bowl, whisk together apple cider vinegar, honey, Dijon mustard, salt, and pepper. Pour the honey dressing over the warm cabbage mixture and toss to combine. Remove from heat and serve immediately.

Approximate Nutritional Value (per serving):

Calories: 90 kcal

Protein: 1g

Fat: 5g

Carbohydrates: 12g

Fiber: 3g

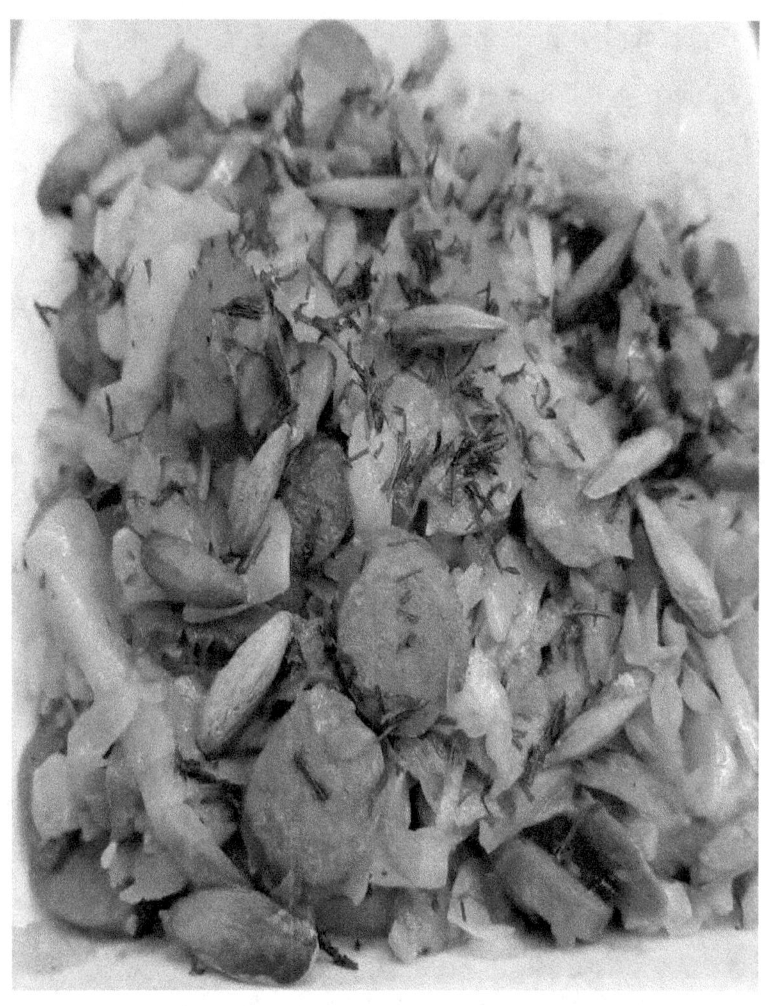

40. Spinach Berry Salad

Ingredients:

4 cups baby spinach leaves

1 cup mixed berries (such as strawberries, blueberries, raspberries)

1/4 cup sliced almonds

2 tablespoons crumbled feta cheese

2 tablespoons balsamic vinaigrette

Preparation Method: In a large bowl, combine baby spinach leaves, mixed berries, sliced almonds, and crumbled feta cheese. Drizzle with balsamic vinaigrette. Toss gently to coat evenly. Serve immediately.

Approximate Nutritional Value (per serving):

Calories: 120 kcal

Protein: 4g

Fat: 8g

Carbohydrates: 10g

Fiber: 4g

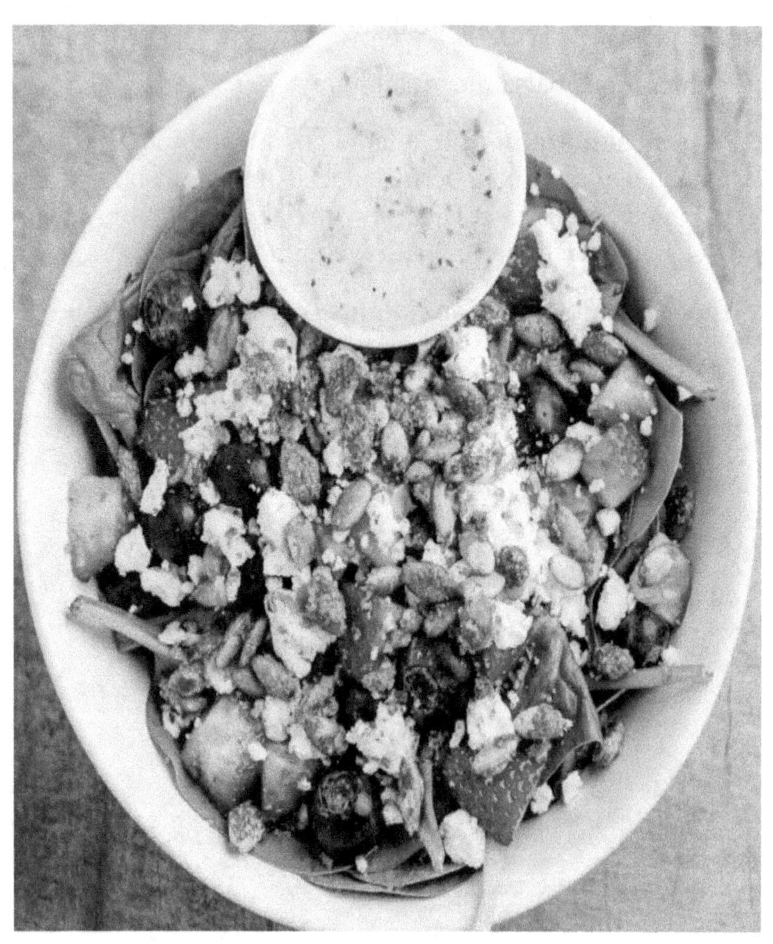

41. Shrimp Apple Salad

Ingredients:

1-pound cooked shrimp, peeled and deveined

2 apples, cored and thinly sliced

1 cup arugula leaves

1/4 cup chopped walnuts

2 tablespoons crumbled blue cheese

2 tablespoons lemon juice

1 tablespoon olive oil

Salt and pepper to taste

Preparation Method: In a large bowl, combine cooked shrimp, sliced apples, arugula leaves, chopped walnuts, and crumbled blue cheese. Drizzle with lemon juice and olive oil. Season with salt and pepper. Toss gently to combine. Serve immediately.

Approximate Nutritional Value (per serving):

Calories: 250 kcal

Protein: 20g

Fat: 12g

Carbohydrates: 18g

Fiber: 4g

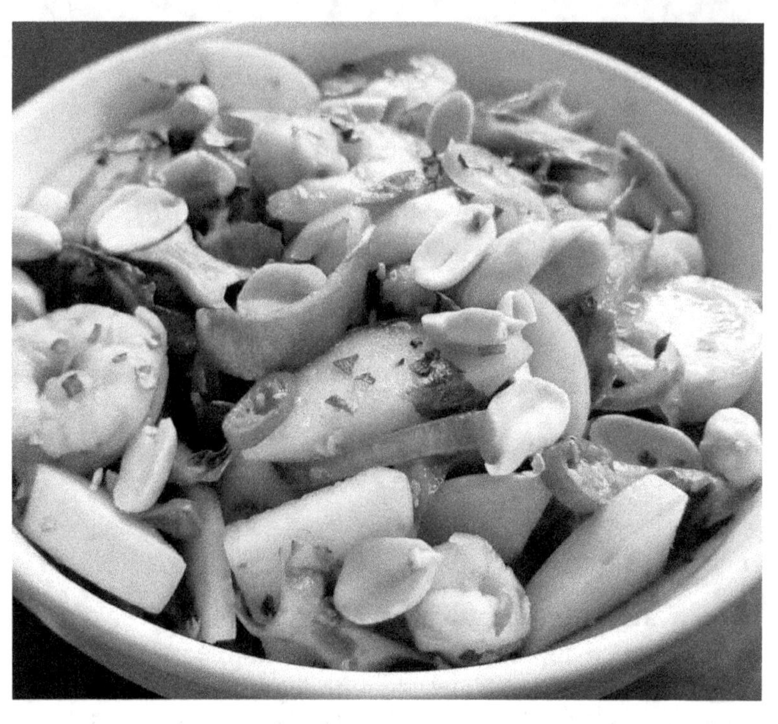

42. Salad Greens with Pears, Fennel, and Walnuts

Ingredients:

4 cups mixed salad greens

2 ripe pears, thinly sliced

1 small fennel bulb, thinly sliced

1/4 cup toasted walnuts

2 tablespoons extra virgin olive oil

1 tablespoon balsamic vinegar

Salt and pepper to taste

Preparation Method: In a large bowl, combine mixed salad greens, sliced pears, sliced fennel, and toasted walnuts. Drizzle with both extra virgin olive oil and balsamic vinegar. Season with salt and pepper. Toss gently to coat evenly. Serve immediately.

Approximate Nutritional Value (per serving):

Calories: 150 kcal

Protein: 2g

Fat: 10g

Carbohydrates: 15g

Fiber: 5g

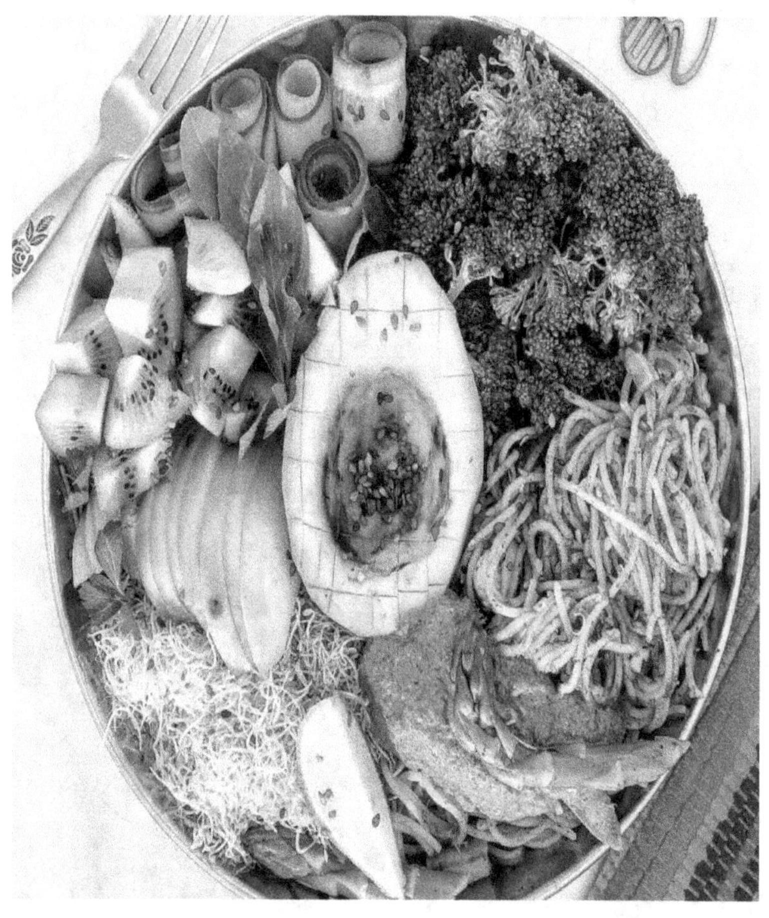

43. Pickled Onion Salad

Ingredients:

1 red onion, thinly sliced

1/4 cup apple cider vinegar

1 tablespoon honey

1/2 teaspoon salt

1/4 teaspoon black pepper

2 cups mixed salad greens

Preparation Method: In a small mixing dish, combine apple cider vinegar, honey, salt, and pepper. Add thinly sliced red onion to the bowl and toss to coat. Let the onions marinate in the vinegar mixture for at least 30 minutes. To serve, arrange mixed salad greens on a plate and top with pickled onions.

Approximate Nutritional Value (per serving):

Calories: 40 kcal

Protein: 1g

Fat: 0g

Carbohydrates: 10g

Fiber: 2g

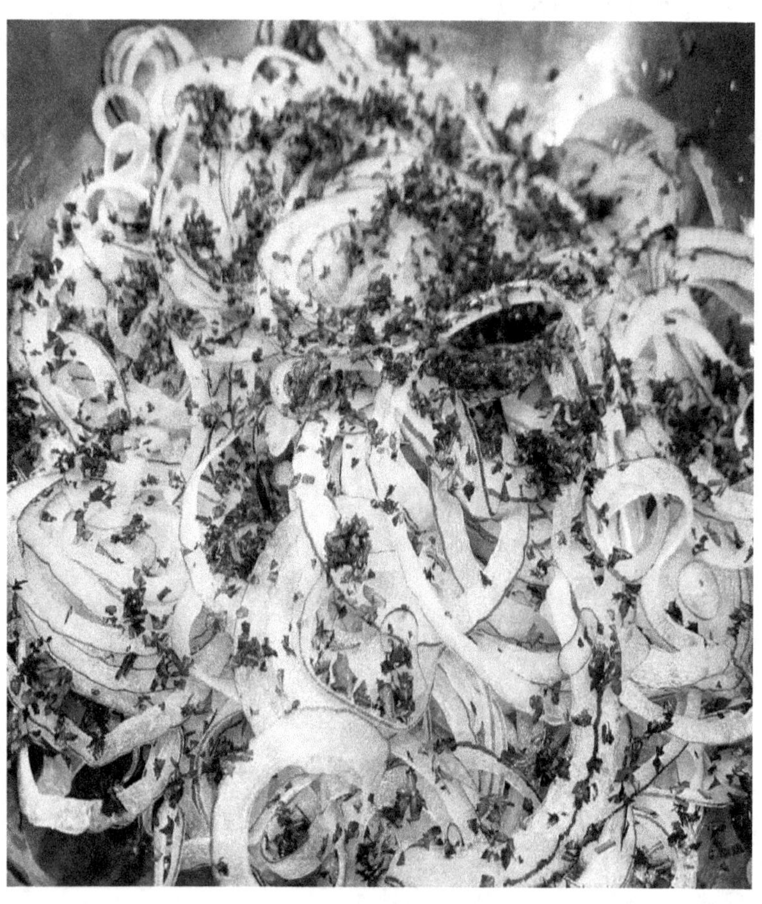

44. French Grilled Lentil Salad

Ingredients:

1 cup cooked green lentils

1/4 cup diced red bell pepper

1/4 cup diced cucumber

2 tablespoons chopped fresh parsley

1 tablespoon chopped fresh mint

2 tablespoons red wine vinegar

1 tablespoon Dijon mustard

2 tablespoons extra virgin olive oil

Salt and pepper to taste

Preparation Method: In a large bowl, combine cooked green lentils, diced red bell pepper, diced cucumber, chopped parsley, and chopped mint. In a small bowl, whisk together red wine vinegar, Dijon mustard, and extra virgin olive oil. Pour the dressing over the lentil mixture and toss to coat. Season with salt and pepper. Serve warm or at room temperature.

Approximate Nutritional Value (per serving):

Calories: 180 kcal

Protein: 8g

Fat: 7g

Carbohydrates: 20g

Fiber: 8g

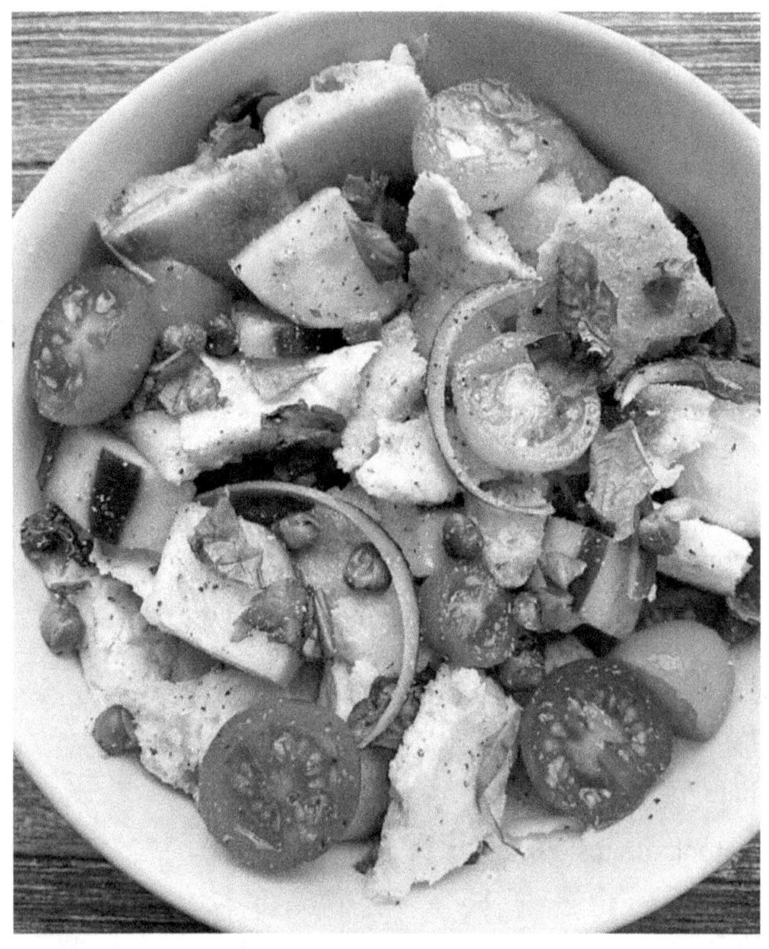

45. English Cucumber Salad with Balsamic Vinaigrette

Ingredients:

2 English cucumbers, thinly sliced

1/4 cup thinly sliced red onion

2 tablespoons chopped fresh dill

2 tablespoons balsamic vinegar

1 tablespoon extra-virgin olive oil

Salt and pepper to taste

Preparation Method: In a large bowl, combine thinly sliced English cucumbers, thinly sliced red onion, and chopped fresh dill. In a small bowl, combine the balsamic vinegar and extra virgin olive oil. Toss the cucumber mixture with the dressing until well coated. Season with salt and pepper. Serve chilled or at room temperature.

Approximate Nutritional Value (per serving):

Calories: 50 kcal

Protein: 1g

Fat: 3g

Carbohydrates: 7g

Fiber: 2g

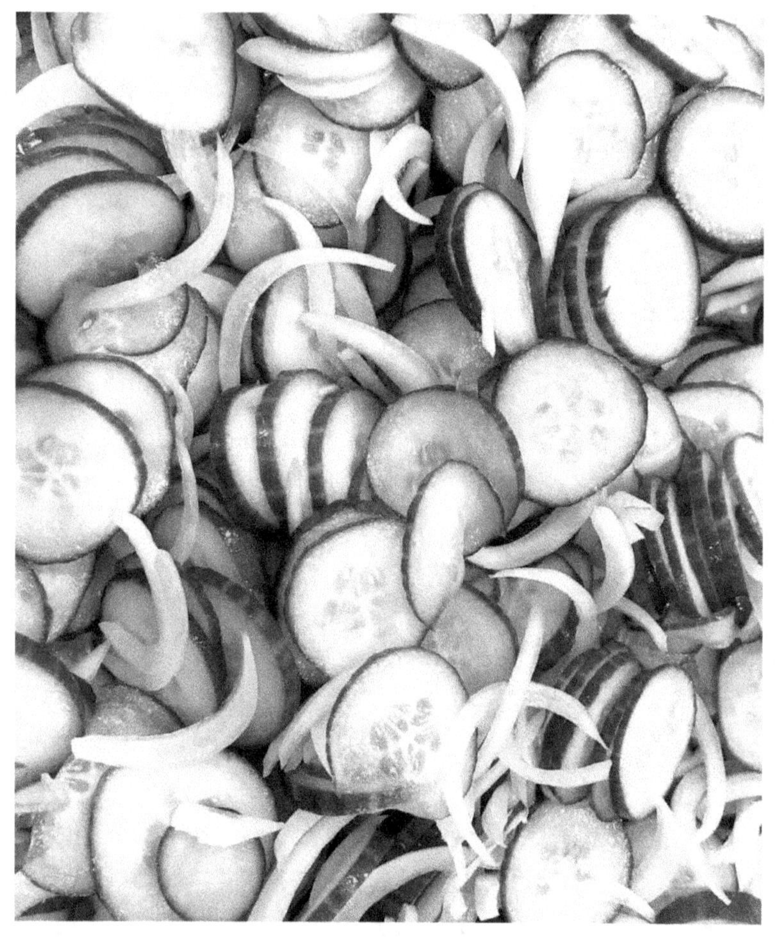

46. Dilled Pasta Salad with Spring Vegetables

Ingredients:

8 oz pasta (such as fusilli or penne)

1 cup cherry tomatoes, halved

1 cup diced cucumber

1/2 cup diced bell pepper

1/4 cup chopped fresh dill

2 tablespoons lemon juice

2 tablespoons extra virgin olive oil

Salt and pepper to taste

Preparation Method: Pasta should be cooked as directed on the package until it is al dente. Drain and rinse under cold water. In a large bowl, combine cooked pasta, cherry tomatoes, diced cucumber, diced bell pepper, and chopped fresh dill. In a small bowl, whisk together lemon juice and extra virgin olive oil. Drizzle the spaghetti mixture with the dressing, then toss to coat. Season with salt and pepper. Serve chilled or at room temperature.

Approximate Nutritional Value (per serving):

Calories: 200 kcal

Protein: 5g

Fat: 6g

Carbohydrates: 30g

Fiber: 3g

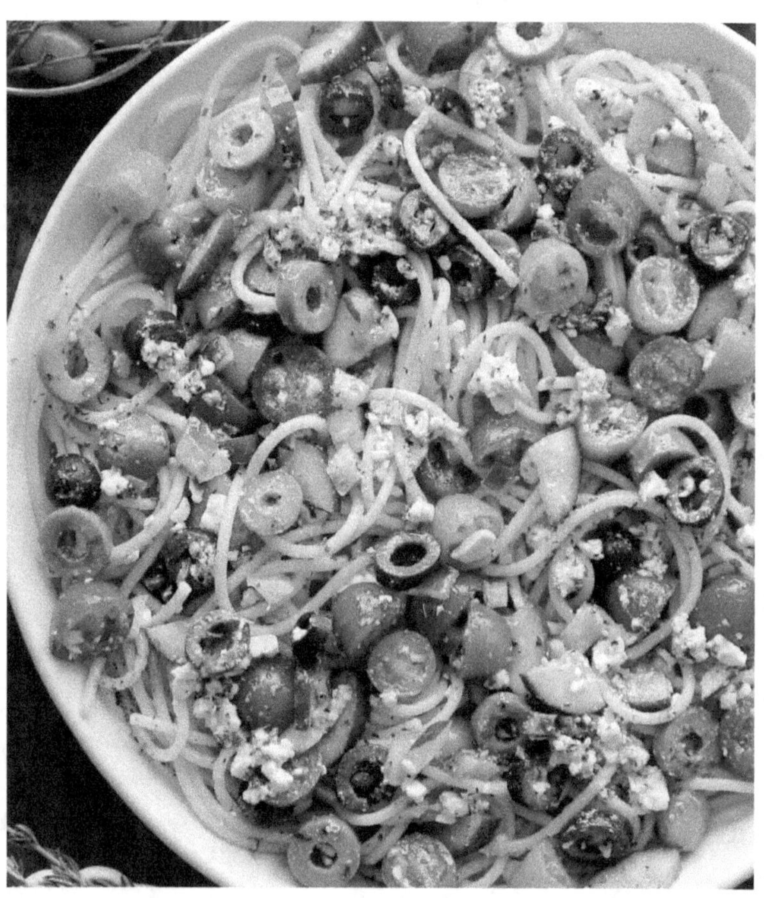

47. Avocado Salad with Ginger Miso Dressing

Ingredients:

2 ripe avocados, diced

2 cups mixed salad greens

1/4 cup shredded carrots

1/4 cup sliced radishes

2 tablespoons chopped fresh cilantro

2 tablespoons rice vinegar

1 tablespoon white miso paste

1 teaspoon grated ginger

1 teaspoon honey

Preparation Method: In a large bowl, combine diced avocados, mixed salad greens, shredded carrots, sliced radishes, and chopped cilantro. In a small bowl, whisk together rice vinegar, white miso paste, grated ginger, honey, sesame oil, salt, and pepper until well combined. Drizzle the salad with the dressing and gently mix to coat. Serve immediately.

Approximate Nutritional Value (per serving):

Calories: 180 kcal

Protein: 3g

Fat: 14g

Carbohydrates: 15g

Fiber: 7g

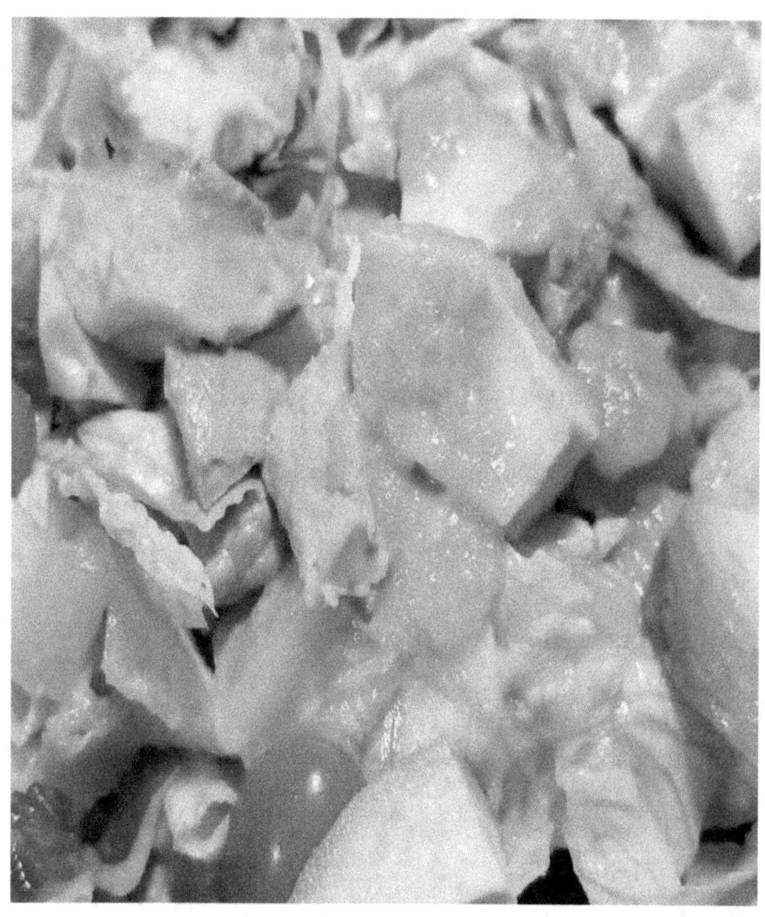

48. Beet Walnut Salad

Ingredients:

4 medium beets, roasted, peeled, and diced

1/2 cup walnuts, toasted and chopped

2 cups mixed salad greens

1/4 cup crumbled goat cheese

2 tablespoons balsamic vinegar

1 tablespoon honey

2 tablespoons extra virgin olive oil

Salt and pepper to taste

Preparation Method: In a large bowl, combine diced roasted beets, chopped walnuts, mixed salad greens, and crumbled goat cheese. In a small bowl, whisk together balsamic vinegar, honey, and extra virgin olive oil. After pouring the dressing over the salad, gently mix to coat. Season with salt and pepper. Serve immediately.

Approximate Nutritional Value (per serving):

Calories: 200 kcal

Protein: 5g

Fat: 15g

Carbohydrates: 15g

Fiber: 4g

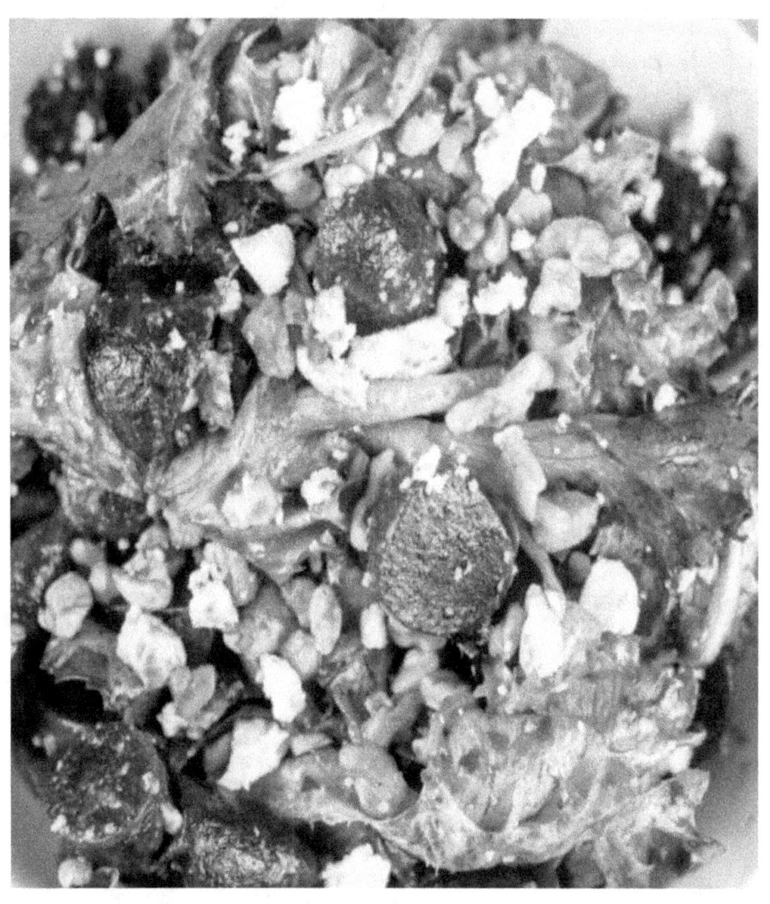

49. Irish Brown Bread

Ingredients:

2 cups whole wheat flour

1 cup all-purpose flour

1 teaspoon baking soda

1/2 teaspoon salt

1 3/4 cups buttermilk

Preparation Method: Preheat the oven to 425°F (220°C) and lightly grease a baking sheet. In a large bowl, sift together whole wheat flour, all-purpose flour, baking soda, and salt. Pour the buttermilk into the well created in the middle of the dry ingredients. Mix with your hands or a wooden spoon until a dough forms. Turn the dough out onto a floured surface and knead lightly until smooth, about 1 minute. Roll the dough into a circular loaf and transfer it to the baking sheet that has been preheated. Make a deep cross on the top of the bread using a sharp knife. Bake for 15 minutes, then reduce the oven temperature to 400°F (200°C) and continue baking for another 20-25 minutes or until the bread is golden brown and sounds hollow when tapped on the bottom. Before slicing, move the bread to a wire rack to cool fully.

Approximate Nutritional Value (per serving - 1 slice):

Calories: 120 kcal

Protein: 4g

Fat: 1g

Carbohydrates: 24g

Fiber: 3g

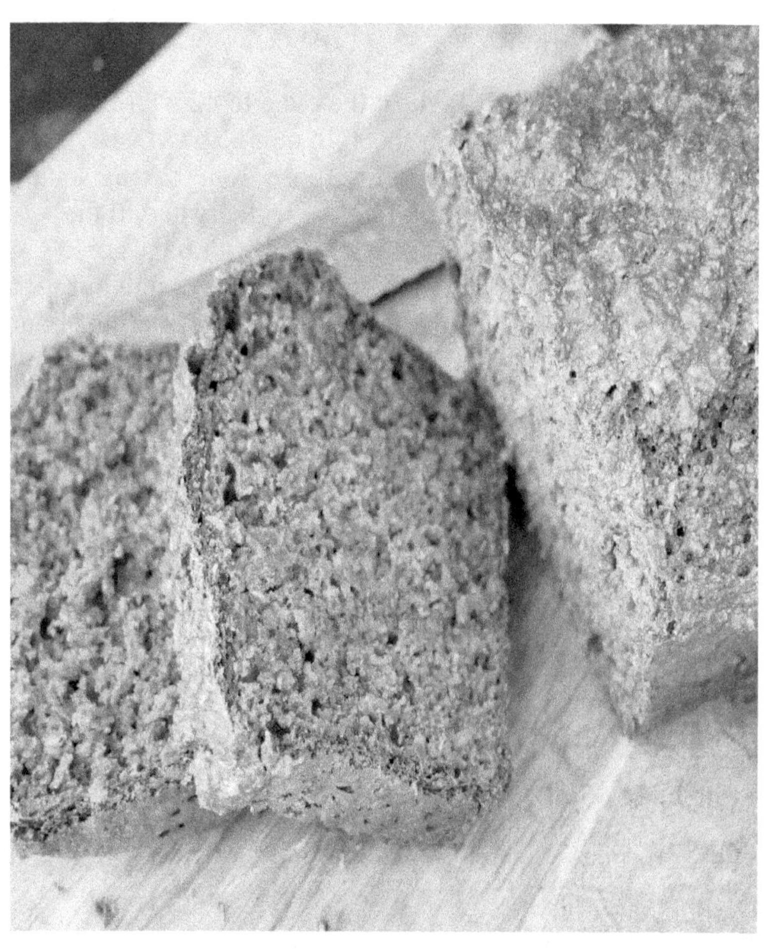

Fiber: 3g

50. Whole-Wheat Soda Bread

Ingredients:

2 cups whole wheat flour

1 cup all-purpose flour

1 teaspoon baking soda

1 teaspoon salt

1 1/4 cups buttermilk

Preparation Method: Preheat the oven to 425°F (220°C) and lightly grease a baking sheet. In a large bowl, sift together whole wheat flour, all-purpose flour, baking soda, and salt. Make a well in the center of the dry ingredients and pour in the buttermilk. Using a wooden spoon or your hands, mix until a dough forms. Turn the dough out onto a floured surface and knead lightly until smooth, about 1 minute. Shape the dough into a round loaf and place it on the prepared baking sheet. Use a sharp knife to score a deep cross on the top of the loaf. Bake for 15 minutes, then reduce the oven temperature to 400°F (200°C) and continue baking for another 20-25 minutes or until the bread is golden brown and sounds hollow when tapped on the bottom. Transfer the bread to a wire rack to cool completely before slicing.

Approximate Nutritional Value (per serving - 1 slice):

Calories: 110 kcal

Protein: 4g

Fat: 1g

Carbohydrates: 22g

Fiber: 3g

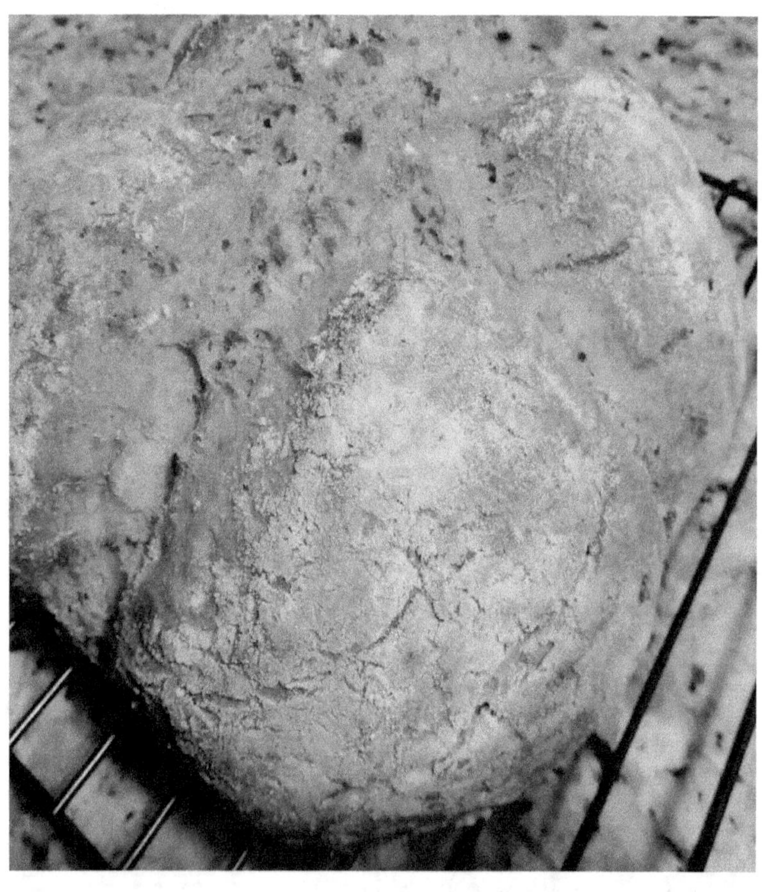

CONCLUSION

"Discovering the delicate balance between managing diabetes and renal health can be daunting for newly diagnosed individuals. However, with the right guidance, it's possible to navigate this journey with confidence and flavor. The cookbook at hand provides a wealth of resources tailored specifically for those facing this dual challenge.

Within its pages, readers will find a treasure trove of carefully curated recipes, each crafted to meet the nutritional needs of diabetic renal patients without sacrificing taste. From nourishing soups to hearty mains and guilt-free desserts, these recipes offer a delicious way to support overall health.

But this cookbook goes beyond mere recipes; it serves as a comprehensive guide to understanding the intricacies of diabetic renal management. Through practical tips on grocery shopping, meal planning, and portion control, individuals can take charge of their health with newfound knowledge and confidence.

In essence, this cookbook isn't just about food; it's about empowerment. It empowers individuals to embrace their dietary requirements, make informed choices, and embark on a journey toward improved health and well-being. With its blend of delicious recipes and invaluable guidance, it's a must-have companion for anyone facing the challenges of diabetes and renal issues."

WEEKLY MEAL PLANNER

MONDAY

BREAKFAST _______________
LUNCH _______________
SNACKS _______________
DINNER _______________

TUESDAY

BREAKFAST _______________
LUNCH _______________
SNACKS _______________
DINNER _______________

WEDNESDAY

BREAKFAST _______________
LUNCH _______________
SNACKS _______________
DINNER _______________

THURSDAY

BREAKFAST _______________
LUNCH _______________
SNACKS _______________
DINNER _______________

FRIDAY

BREAKFAST _______________
LUNCH _______________
SNACKS _______________
DINNER _______________

SATURDAY

BREAKFAST _______________
LUNCH _______________
SNACKS _______________
DINNER _______________

SUNDAY

BREAKFAST _______________
LUNCH _______________
SNACKS _______________
DINNER _______________

NOTES

____
____
____
____

WEEKLY MEAL PLANNER

MONDAY

BREAKFAST ______________________

LUNCH ______________________

SNACKS ______________________

DINNER ______________________

TUESDAY

BREAKFAST ______________________

LUNCH ______________________

SNACKS ______________________

DINNER ______________________

WEDNESDAY

BREAKFAST ______________________

LUNCH ______________________

SNACKS ______________________

DINNER ______________________

THURSDAY

BREAKFAST ______________________

LUNCH ______________________

SNACKS ______________________

DINNER ______________________

FRIDAY

BREAKFAST ______________________

LUNCH ______________________

SNACKS ______________________

DINNER ______________________

SATURDAY

BREAKFAST ______________________

LUNCH ______________________

SNACKS ______________________

DINNER ______________________

SUNDAY

BREAKFAST ______________________

LUNCH ______________________

SNACKS ______________________

DINNER ______________________

NOTES

____

____

____

____

WEEKLY MEAL PLANNER

MONDAY

BREAKFAST _______________

LUNCH _______________

SNACKS _______________

DINNER _______________

TUESDAY

BREAKFAST _______________

LUNCH _______________

SNACKS _______________

DINNER _______________

WEDNESDAY

BREAKFAST _______________

LUNCH _______________

SNACKS _______________

DINNER _______________

THURSDAY

BREAKFAST _______________

LUNCH _______________

SNACKS _______________

DINNER _______________

FRIDAY

BREAKFAST _______________

LUNCH _______________

SNACKS _______________

DINNER _______________

SATURDAY

BREAKFAST _______________

LUNCH _______________

SNACKS _______________

DINNER _______________

SUNDAY

BREAKFAST _______________

LUNCH _______________

SNACKS _______________

DINNER _______________

NOTES

____

____

____

____

WEEKLY MEAL PLANNER

MONDAY

BREAKFAST ___________________

LUNCH ___________________

SNACKS ___________________

DINNER ___________________

TUESDAY

BREAKFAST ___________________

LUNCH ___________________

SNACKS ___________________

DINNER ___________________

WEDNESDAY

BREAKFAST ___________________

LUNCH ___________________

SNACKS ___________________

DINNER ___________________

THURSDAY

BREAKFAST ___________________

LUNCH ___________________

SNACKS ___________________

DINNER ___________________

FRIDAY

BREAKFAST ___________________

LUNCH ___________________

SNACKS ___________________

DINNER ___________________

SATURDAY

BREAKFAST ___________________

LUNCH ___________________

SNACKS ___________________

DINNER ___________________

SUNDAY

BREAKFAST ___________________

LUNCH ___________________

SNACKS ___________________

DINNER ___________________

NOTES

____

____

____

____

WEEKLY MEAL PLANNER

MONDAY

BREAKFAST ___________________

LUNCH ___________________

SNACKS ___________________

DINNER ___________________

TUESDAY

BREAKFAST ___________________

LUNCH ___________________

SNACKS ___________________

DINNER ___________________

WEDNESDAY

BREAKFAST ___________________

LUNCH ___________________

SNACKS ___________________

DINNER ___________________

THURSDAY

BREAKFAST ___________________

LUNCH ___________________

SNACKS ___________________

DINNER ___________________

FRIDAY

BREAKFAST ___________________

LUNCH ___________________

SNACKS ___________________

DINNER ___________________

SATURDAY

BREAKFAST ___________________

LUNCH ___________________

SNACKS ___________________

DINNER ___________________

SUNDAY

BREAKFAST ___________________

LUNCH ___________________

SNACKS ___________________

DINNER ___________________

NOTES

____

____

____

____

WEEKLY MEAL PLANNER

MONDAY

BREAKFAST ______________________

LUNCH ______________________

SNACKS ______________________

DINNER ______________________

TUESDAY

BREAKFAST ______________________

LUNCH ______________________

SNACKS ______________________

DINNER ______________________

WEDNESDAY

BREAKFAST ______________________

LUNCH ______________________

SNACKS ______________________

DINNER ______________________

THURSDAY

BREAKFAST ______________________

LUNCH ______________________

SNACKS ______________________

DINNER ______________________

FRIDAY

BREAKFAST ______________________

LUNCH ______________________

SNACKS ______________________

DINNER ______________________

SATURDAY

BREAKFAST ______________________

LUNCH ______________________

SNACKS ______________________

DINNER ______________________

SUNDAY

BREAKFAST ______________________

LUNCH ______________________

SNACKS ______________________

DINNER ______________________

NOTES

____

____

____

____

WEEKLY MEAL PLANNER

MONDAY

BREAKFAST __________________

LUNCH __________________

SNACKS __________________

DINNER __________________

TUESDAY

BREAKFAST __________________

LUNCH __________________

SNACKS __________________

DINNER __________________

WEDNESDAY

BREAKFAST __________________

LUNCH __________________

SNACKS __________________

DINNER __________________

THURSDAY

BREAKFAST __________________

LUNCH __________________

SNACKS __________________

DINNER __________________

FRIDAY

BREAKFAST __________________

LUNCH __________________

SNACKS __________________

DINNER __________________

SATURDAY

BREAKFAST __________________

LUNCH __________________

SNACKS __________________

DINNER __________________

SUNDAY

BREAKFAST __________________

LUNCH __________________

SNACKS __________________

DINNER __________________

NOTES

____

____

____

____

WEEKLY MEAL PLANNER

MONDAY

BREAKFAST _______________

LUNCH _______________

SNACKS _______________

DINNER _______________

TUESDAY

BREAKFAST _______________

LUNCH _______________

SNACKS _______________

DINNER _______________

WEDNESDAY

BREAKFAST _______________

LUNCH _______________

SNACKS _______________

DINNER _______________

THURSDAY

BREAKFAST _______________

LUNCH _______________

SNACKS _______________

DINNER _______________

FRIDAY

BREAKFAST _______________

LUNCH _______________

SNACKS _______________

DINNER _______________

SATURDAY

BREAKFAST _______________

LUNCH _______________

SNACKS _______________

DINNER _______________

SUNDAY

BREAKFAST _______________

LUNCH _______________

SNACKS _______________

DINNER _______________

NOTES

____

____

____

____

WEEKLY MEAL PLANNER

MONDAY

BREAKFAST __________

LUNCH __________

SNACKS __________

DINNER __________

TUESDAY

BREAKFAST __________

LUNCH __________

SNACKS __________

DINNER __________

WEDNESDAY

BREAKFAST __________

LUNCH __________

SNACKS __________

DINNER __________

THURSDAY

BREAKFAST __________

LUNCH __________

SNACKS __________

DINNER __________

FRIDAY

BREAKFAST __________

LUNCH __________

SNACKS __________

DINNER __________

SATURDAY

BREAKFAST __________

LUNCH __________

SNACKS __________

DINNER __________

SUNDAY

BREAKFAST __________

LUNCH __________

SNACKS __________

DINNER __________

NOTES

WEEKLY MEAL PLANNER

MONDAY

BREAKFAST ___________________

LUNCH ___________________

SNACKS ___________________

DINNER ___________________

TUESDAY

BREAKFAST ___________________

LUNCH ___________________

SNACKS ___________________

DINNER ___________________

WEDNESDAY

BREAKFAST ___________________

LUNCH ___________________

SNACKS ___________________

DINNER ___________________

THURSDAY

BREAKFAST ___________________

LUNCH ___________________

SNACKS ___________________

DINNER ___________________

FRIDAY

BREAKFAST ___________________

LUNCH ___________________

SNACKS ___________________

DINNER ___________________

SATURDAY

BREAKFAST ___________________

LUNCH ___________________

SNACKS ___________________

DINNER ___________________

SUNDAY

BREAKFAST ___________________

LUNCH ___________________

SNACKS ___________________

DINNER ___________________

NOTES

____

____

____

____

WEEKLY MEAL PLANNER

MONDAY

BREAKFAST __________________

LUNCH __________________

SNACKS __________________

DINNER __________________

TUESDAY

BREAKFAST __________________

LUNCH __________________

SNACKS __________________

DINNER __________________

WEDNESDAY

BREAKFAST __________________

LUNCH __________________

SNACKS __________________

DINNER __________________

THURSDAY

BREAKFAST __________________

LUNCH __________________

SNACKS __________________

DINNER __________________

FRIDAY

BREAKFAST __________________

LUNCH __________________

SNACKS __________________

DINNER __________________

SATURDAY

BREAKFAST __________________

LUNCH __________________

SNACKS __________________

DINNER __________________

SUNDAY

BREAKFAST __________________

LUNCH __________________

SNACKS __________________

DINNER __________________

NOTES

____

____

____

____

WEEKLY MEAL PLANNER

MONDAY

BREAKFAST __________________

LUNCH __________________

SNACKS __________________

DINNER __________________

TUESDAY

BREAKFAST __________________

LUNCH __________________

SNACKS __________________

DINNER __________________

WEDNESDAY

BREAKFAST __________________

LUNCH __________________

SNACKS __________________

DINNER __________________

THURSDAY

BREAKFAST __________________

LUNCH __________________

SNACKS __________________

DINNER __________________

FRIDAY

BREAKFAST __________________

LUNCH __________________

SNACKS __________________

DINNER __________________

SATURDAY

BREAKFAST __________________

LUNCH __________________

SNACKS __________________

DINNER __________________

SUNDAY

BREAKFAST __________________

LUNCH __________________

SNACKS __________________

DINNER __________________

NOTES

____

____

____

____

WEEKLY MEAL PLANNER

MONDAY

BREAKFAST _______________

LUNCH _______________

SNACKS _______________

DINNER _______________

TUESDAY

BREAKFAST _______________

LUNCH _______________

SNACKS _______________

DINNER _______________

WEDNESDAY

BREAKFAST _______________

LUNCH _______________

SNACKS _______________

DINNER _______________

THURSDAY

BREAKFAST _______________

LUNCH _______________

SNACKS _______________

DINNER _______________

FRIDAY

BREAKFAST _______________

LUNCH _______________

SNACKS _______________

DINNER _______________

SATURDAY

BREAKFAST _______________

LUNCH _______________

SNACKS _______________

DINNER _______________

SUNDAY

BREAKFAST _______________

LUNCH _______________

SNACKS _______________

DINNER _______________

NOTES

____

____

____

____

WEEKLY MEAL PLANNER

MONDAY

BREAKFAST ___________________

LUNCH ___________________

SNACKS ___________________

DINNER ___________________

TUESDAY

BREAKFAST ___________________

LUNCH ___________________

SNACKS ___________________

DINNER ___________________

WEDNESDAY

BREAKFAST ___________________

LUNCH ___________________

SNACKS ___________________

DINNER ___________________

THURSDAY

BREAKFAST ___________________

LUNCH ___________________

SNACKS ___________________

DINNER ___________________

FRIDAY

BREAKFAST ___________________

LUNCH ___________________

SNACKS ___________________

DINNER ___________________

SATURDAY

BREAKFAST ___________________

LUNCH ___________________

SNACKS ___________________

DINNER ___________________

SUNDAY

BREAKFAST ___________________

LUNCH ___________________

SNACKS ___________________

DINNER ___________________

NOTES

____

____

____

____

WEEKLY MEAL PLANNER

MONDAY

BREAKFAST ___________________

LUNCH ___________________

SNACKS ___________________

DINNER ___________________

TUESDAY

BREAKFAST ___________________

LUNCH ___________________

SNACKS ___________________

DINNER ___________________

WEDNESDAY

BREAKFAST ___________________

LUNCH ___________________

SNACKS ___________________

DINNER ___________________

THURSDAY

BREAKFAST ___________________

LUNCH ___________________

SNACKS ___________________

DINNER ___________________

FRIDAY

BREAKFAST ___________________

LUNCH ___________________

SNACKS ___________________

DINNER ___________________

SATURDAY

BREAKFAST ___________________

LUNCH ___________________

SNACKS ___________________

DINNER ___________________

SUNDAY

BREAKFAST ___________________

LUNCH ___________________

SNACKS ___________________

DINNER ___________________

NOTES

____

____

____

____

WEEKLY MEAL PLANNER

MONDAY

BREAKFAST _______________________

LUNCH _______________________

SNACKS _______________________

DINNER _______________________

TUESDAY

BREAKFAST _______________________

LUNCH _______________________

SNACKS _______________________

DINNER _______________________

WEDNESDAY

BREAKFAST _______________________

LUNCH _______________________

SNACKS _______________________

DINNER _______________________

THURSDAY

BREAKFAST _______________________

LUNCH _______________________

SNACKS _______________________

DINNER _______________________

FRIDAY

BREAKFAST _______________________

LUNCH _______________________

SNACKS _______________________

DINNER _______________________

SATURDAY

BREAKFAST _______________________

LUNCH _______________________

SNACKS _______________________

DINNER _______________________

SUNDAY

BREAKFAST _______________________

LUNCH _______________________

SNACKS _______________________

DINNER _______________________

NOTES

____

____

____

____

WEEKLY MEAL PLANNER

MONDAY

BREAKFAST ______________________

LUNCH ______________________

SNACKS ______________________

DINNER ______________________

TUESDAY

BREAKFAST ______________________

LUNCH ______________________

SNACKS ______________________

DINNER ______________________

WEDNESDAY

BREAKFAST ______________________

LUNCH ______________________

SNACKS ______________________

DINNER ______________________

THURSDAY

BREAKFAST ______________________

LUNCH ______________________

SNACKS ______________________

DINNER ______________________

FRIDAY

BREAKFAST ______________________

LUNCH ______________________

SNACKS ______________________

DINNER ______________________

SATURDAY

BREAKFAST ______________________

LUNCH ______________________

SNACKS ______________________

DINNER ______________________

SUNDAY

BREAKFAST ______________________

LUNCH ______________________

SNACKS ______________________

DINNER ______________________

NOTES

____

____

____

____

WEEKLY MEAL PLANNER

MONDAY

BREAKFAST _______________

LUNCH _______________

SNACKS _______________

DINNER _______________

TUESDAY

BREAKFAST _______________

LUNCH _______________

SNACKS _______________

DINNER _______________

WEDNESDAY

BREAKFAST _______________

LUNCH _______________

SNACKS _______________

DINNER _______________

THURSDAY

BREAKFAST _______________

LUNCH _______________

SNACKS _______________

DINNER _______________

FRIDAY

BREAKFAST _______________

LUNCH _______________

SNACKS _______________

DINNER _______________

SATURDAY

BREAKFAST _______________

LUNCH _______________

SNACKS _______________

DINNER _______________

SUNDAY

BREAKFAST _______________

LUNCH _______________

SNACKS _______________

DINNER _______________

NOTES

____

____

____

____

WEEKLY MEAL PLANNER

MONDAY

BREAKFAST ___________________

LUNCH ___________________

SNACKS ___________________

DINNER ___________________

TUESDAY

BREAKFAST ___________________

LUNCH ___________________

SNACKS ___________________

DINNER ___________________

WEDNESDAY

BREAKFAST ___________________

LUNCH ___________________

SNACKS ___________________

DINNER ___________________

THURSDAY

BREAKFAST ___________________

LUNCH ___________________

SNACKS ___________________

DINNER ___________________

FRIDAY

BREAKFAST ___________________

LUNCH ___________________

SNACKS ___________________

DINNER ___________________

SATURDAY

BREAKFAST ___________________

LUNCH ___________________

SNACKS ___________________

DINNER ___________________

SUNDAY

BREAKFAST ___________________

LUNCH ___________________

SNACKS ___________________

DINNER ___________________

NOTES

____

____

____

WEEKLY MEAL PLANNER

MONDAY

BREAKFAST ___________________

LUNCH ___________________

SNACKS ___________________

DINNER ___________________

TUESDAY

BREAKFAST ___________________

LUNCH ___________________

SNACKS ___________________

DINNER ___________________

WEDNESDAY

BREAKFAST ___________________

LUNCH ___________________

SNACKS ___________________

DINNER ___________________

THURSDAY

BREAKFAST ___________________

LUNCH ___________________

SNACKS ___________________

DINNER ___________________

FRIDAY

BREAKFAST ___________________

LUNCH ___________________

SNACKS ___________________

DINNER ___________________

SATURDAY

BREAKFAST ___________________

LUNCH ___________________

SNACKS ___________________

DINNER ___________________

SUNDAY

BREAKFAST ___________________

LUNCH ___________________

SNACKS ___________________

DINNER ___________________

NOTES

____

____

____

____

WEEKLY MEAL PLANNER

MONDAY

BREAKFAST _______________
LUNCH _______________
SNACKS _______________
DINNER _______________

TUESDAY

BREAKFAST _______________
LUNCH _______________
SNACKS _______________
DINNER _______________

WEDNESDAY

BREAKFAST _______________
LUNCH _______________
SNACKS _______________
DINNER _______________

THURSDAY

BREAKFAST _______________
LUNCH _______________
SNACKS _______________
DINNER _______________

FRIDAY

BREAKFAST _______________
LUNCH _______________
SNACKS _______________
DINNER _______________

SATURDAY

BREAKFAST _______________
LUNCH _______________
SNACKS _______________
DINNER _______________

SUNDAY

BREAKFAST _______________
LUNCH _______________
SNACKS _______________
DINNER _______________

NOTES

____
____
____
____

WEEKLY MEAL PLANNER

MONDAY

BREAKFAST ______________________

LUNCH ______________________

SNACKS ______________________

DINNER ______________________

TUESDAY

BREAKFAST ______________________

LUNCH ______________________

SNACKS ______________________

DINNER ______________________

WEDNESDAY

BREAKFAST ______________________

LUNCH ______________________

SNACKS ______________________

DINNER ______________________

THURSDAY

BREAKFAST ______________________

LUNCH ______________________

SNACKS ______________________

DINNER ______________________

FRIDAY

BREAKFAST ______________________

LUNCH ______________________

SNACKS ______________________

DINNER ______________________

SATURDAY

BREAKFAST ______________________

LUNCH ______________________

SNACKS ______________________

DINNER ______________________

SUNDAY

BREAKFAST ______________________

LUNCH ______________________

SNACKS ______________________

DINNER ______________________

NOTES

____

____

____

____

WEEKLY MEAL PLANNER

MONDAY

BREAKFAST _______________

LUNCH _______________

SNACKS _______________

DINNER _______________

TUESDAY

BREAKFAST _______________

LUNCH _______________

SNACKS _______________

DINNER _______________

WEDNESDAY

BREAKFAST _______________

LUNCH _______________

SNACKS _______________

DINNER _______________

THURSDAY

BREAKFAST _______________

LUNCH _______________

SNACKS _______________

DINNER _______________

FRIDAY

BREAKFAST _______________

LUNCH _______________

SNACKS _______________

DINNER _______________

SATURDAY

BREAKFAST _______________

LUNCH _______________

SNACKS _______________

DINNER _______________

SUNDAY

BREAKFAST _______________

LUNCH _______________

SNACKS _______________

DINNER _______________

NOTES

____

____

____

____

WEEKLY MEAL PLANNER

MONDAY

BREAKFAST _______________

LUNCH _______________

SNACKS _______________

DINNER _______________

TUESDAY

BREAKFAST _______________

LUNCH _______________

SNACKS _______________

DINNER _______________

WEDNESDAY

BREAKFAST _______________

LUNCH _______________

SNACKS _______________

DINNER _______________

THURSDAY

BREAKFAST _______________

LUNCH _______________

SNACKS _______________

DINNER _______________

FRIDAY

BREAKFAST _______________

LUNCH _______________

SNACKS _______________

DINNER _______________

SATURDAY

BREAKFAST _______________

LUNCH _______________

SNACKS _______________

DINNER _______________

SUNDAY

BREAKFAST _______________

LUNCH _______________

SNACKS _______________

DINNER _______________

NOTES

____

____

____

____

WEEKLY MEAL PLANNER

MONDAY

BREAKFAST _______________

LUNCH _______________

SNACKS _______________

DINNER _______________

TUESDAY

BREAKFAST _______________

LUNCH _______________

SNACKS _______________

DINNER _______________

WEDNESDAY

BREAKFAST _______________

LUNCH _______________

SNACKS _______________

DINNER _______________

THURSDAY

BREAKFAST _______________

LUNCH _______________

SNACKS _______________

DINNER _______________

FRIDAY

BREAKFAST _______________

LUNCH _______________

SNACKS _______________

DINNER _______________

SATURDAY

BREAKFAST _______________

LUNCH _______________

SNACKS _______________

DINNER _______________

SUNDAY

BREAKFAST _______________

LUNCH _______________

SNACKS _______________

DINNER _______________

NOTES

____

____

____

____

WEEKLY MEAL PLANNER

MONDAY

BREAKFAST __________________

LUNCH _____________________

SNACKS ____________________

DINNER ____________________

TUESDAY

BREAKFAST __________________

LUNCH _____________________

SNACKS ____________________

DINNER ____________________

WEDNESDAY

BREAKFAST __________________

LUNCH _____________________

SNACKS ____________________

DINNER ____________________

THURSDAY

BREAKFAST __________________

LUNCH _____________________

SNACKS ____________________

DINNER ____________________

FRIDAY

BREAKFAST __________________

LUNCH _____________________

SNACKS ____________________

DINNER ____________________

SATURDAY

BREAKFAST __________________

LUNCH _____________________

SNACKS ____________________

DINNER ____________________

SUNDAY

BREAKFAST __________________

LUNCH _____________________

SNACKS ____________________

DINNER ____________________

NOTES

____

____

____

____

WEEKLY MEAL PLANNER

MONDAY

BREAKFAST ___________________

LUNCH ___________________

SNACKS ___________________

DINNER ___________________

TUESDAY

BREAKFAST ___________________

LUNCH ___________________

SNACKS ___________________

DINNER ___________________

WEDNESDAY

BREAKFAST ___________________

LUNCH ___________________

SNACKS ___________________

DINNER ___________________

THURSDAY

BREAKFAST ___________________

LUNCH ___________________

SNACKS ___________________

DINNER ___________________

FRIDAY

BREAKFAST ___________________

LUNCH ___________________

SNACKS ___________________

DINNER ___________________

SATURDAY

BREAKFAST ___________________

LUNCH ___________________

SNACKS ___________________

DINNER ___________________

SUNDAY

BREAKFAST ___________________

LUNCH ___________________

SNACKS ___________________

DINNER ___________________

NOTES

____

____

____

WEEKLY MEAL PLANNER

MONDAY

BREAKFAST ___________________

LUNCH ___________________

SNACKS ___________________

DINNER ___________________

TUESDAY

BREAKFAST ___________________

LUNCH ___________________

SNACKS ___________________

DINNER ___________________

WEDNESDAY

BREAKFAST ___________________

LUNCH ___________________

SNACKS ___________________

DINNER ___________________

THURSDAY

BREAKFAST ___________________

LUNCH ___________________

SNACKS ___________________

DINNER ___________________

FRIDAY

BREAKFAST ___________________

LUNCH ___________________

SNACKS ___________________

DINNER ___________________

SATURDAY

BREAKFAST ___________________

LUNCH ___________________

SNACKS ___________________

DINNER ___________________

SUNDAY

BREAKFAST ___________________

LUNCH ___________________

SNACKS ___________________

DINNER ___________________

NOTES

____

____

____

____

WEEKLY MEAL PLANNER

MONDAY

BREAKFAST ___________________

LUNCH ___________________

SNACKS ___________________

DINNER ___________________

TUESDAY

BREAKFAST ___________________

LUNCH ___________________

SNACKS ___________________

DINNER ___________________

WEDNESDAY

BREAKFAST ___________________

LUNCH ___________________

SNACKS ___________________

DINNER ___________________

THURSDAY

BREAKFAST ___________________

LUNCH ___________________

SNACKS ___________________

DINNER ___________________

FRIDAY

BREAKFAST ___________________

LUNCH ___________________

SNACKS ___________________

DINNER ___________________

SATURDAY

BREAKFAST ___________________

LUNCH ___________________

SNACKS ___________________

DINNER ___________________

SUNDAY

BREAKFAST ___________________

LUNCH ___________________

SNACKS ___________________

DINNER ___________________

NOTES

____

____

____

____

WEEKLY MEAL PLANNER

MONDAY

BREAKFAST _______________________

LUNCH _______________________

SNACKS _______________________

DINNER _______________________

TUESDAY

BREAKFAST _______________________

LUNCH _______________________

SNACKS _______________________

DINNER _______________________

WEDNESDAY

BREAKFAST _______________________

LUNCH _______________________

SNACKS _______________________

DINNER _______________________

THURSDAY

BREAKFAST _______________________

LUNCH _______________________

SNACKS _______________________

DINNER _______________________

FRIDAY

BREAKFAST _______________________

LUNCH _______________________

SNACKS _______________________

DINNER _______________________

SATURDAY

BREAKFAST _______________________

LUNCH _______________________

SNACKS _______________________

DINNER _______________________

SUNDAY

BREAKFAST _______________________

LUNCH _______________________

SNACKS _______________________

DINNER _______________________

NOTES

____

____

____

____

WEEKLY MEAL PLANNER

MONDAY

BREAKFAST ___________________

LUNCH ___________________

SNACKS ___________________

DINNER ___________________

TUESDAY

BREAKFAST ___________________

LUNCH ___________________

SNACKS ___________________

DINNER ___________________

WEDNESDAY

BREAKFAST ___________________

LUNCH ___________________

SNACKS ___________________

DINNER ___________________

THURSDAY

BREAKFAST ___________________

LUNCH ___________________

SNACKS ___________________

DINNER ___________________

FRIDAY

BREAKFAST ___________________

LUNCH ___________________

SNACKS ___________________

DINNER ___________________

SATURDAY

BREAKFAST ___________________

LUNCH ___________________

SNACKS ___________________

DINNER ___________________

SUNDAY

BREAKFAST ___________________

LUNCH ___________________

SNACKS ___________________

DINNER ___________________

NOTES

____

____

____

____

WEEKLY MEAL PLANNER

MONDAY

BREAKFAST ______________________
LUNCH ______________________
SNACKS ______________________
DINNER ______________________

TUESDAY

BREAKFAST ______________________
LUNCH ______________________
SNACKS ______________________
DINNER ______________________

WEDNESDAY

BREAKFAST ______________________
LUNCH ______________________
SNACKS ______________________
DINNER ______________________

THURSDAY

BREAKFAST ______________________
LUNCH ______________________
SNACKS ______________________
DINNER ______________________

FRIDAY

BREAKFAST ______________________
LUNCH ______________________
SNACKS ______________________
DINNER ______________________

SATURDAY

BREAKFAST ______________________
LUNCH ______________________
SNACKS ______________________
DINNER ______________________

SUNDAY

BREAKFAST ______________________
LUNCH ______________________
SNACKS ______________________
DINNER ______________________

NOTES

____
____
____
____

WEEKLY MEAL PLANNER

MONDAY

BREAKFAST _______________

LUNCH _______________

SNACKS _______________

DINNER _______________

TUESDAY

BREAKFAST _______________

LUNCH _______________

SNACKS _______________

DINNER _______________

WEDNESDAY

BREAKFAST _______________

LUNCH _______________

SNACKS _______________

DINNER _______________

THURSDAY

BREAKFAST _______________

LUNCH _______________

SNACKS _______________

DINNER _______________

FRIDAY

BREAKFAST _______________

LUNCH _______________

SNACKS _______________

DINNER _______________

SATURDAY

BREAKFAST _______________

LUNCH _______________

SNACKS _______________

DINNER _______________

SUNDAY

BREAKFAST _______________

LUNCH _______________

SNACKS _______________

DINNER _______________

NOTES

____

____

____

____

WEEKLY MEAL PLANNER

MONDAY

BREAKFAST __________________

LUNCH __________________

SNACKS __________________

DINNER __________________

TUESDAY

BREAKFAST __________________

LUNCH __________________

SNACKS __________________

DINNER __________________

WEDNESDAY

BREAKFAST __________________

LUNCH __________________

SNACKS __________________

DINNER __________________

THURSDAY

BREAKFAST __________________

LUNCH __________________

SNACKS __________________

DINNER __________________

FRIDAY

BREAKFAST __________________

LUNCH __________________

SNACKS __________________

DINNER __________________

SATURDAY

BREAKFAST __________________

LUNCH __________________

SNACKS __________________

DINNER __________________

SUNDAY

BREAKFAST __________________

LUNCH __________________

SNACKS __________________

DINNER __________________

NOTES

____

____

____

____

WEEKLY MEAL PLANNER

MONDAY

BREAKFAST __________________

LUNCH __________________

SNACKS __________________

DINNER __________________

TUESDAY

BREAKFAST __________________

LUNCH __________________

SNACKS __________________

DINNER __________________

WEDNESDAY

BREAKFAST __________________

LUNCH __________________

SNACKS __________________

DINNER __________________

THURSDAY

BREAKFAST __________________

LUNCH __________________

SNACKS __________________

DINNER __________________

FRIDAY

BREAKFAST __________________

LUNCH __________________

SNACKS __________________

DINNER __________________

SATURDAY

BREAKFAST __________________

LUNCH __________________

SNACKS __________________

DINNER __________________

SUNDAY

BREAKFAST __________________

LUNCH __________________

SNACKS __________________

DINNER __________________

NOTES

____

____

____

____

WEEKLY MEAL PLANNER

MONDAY

BREAKFAST ___________________

LUNCH ___________________

SNACKS ___________________

DINNER ___________________

TUESDAY

BREAKFAST ___________________

LUNCH ___________________

SNACKS ___________________

DINNER ___________________

WEDNESDAY

BREAKFAST ___________________

LUNCH ___________________

SNACKS ___________________

DINNER ___________________

THURSDAY

BREAKFAST ___________________

LUNCH ___________________

SNACKS ___________________

DINNER ___________________

FRIDAY

BREAKFAST ___________________

LUNCH ___________________

SNACKS ___________________

DINNER ___________________

SATURDAY

BREAKFAST ___________________

LUNCH ___________________

SNACKS ___________________

DINNER ___________________

SUNDAY

BREAKFAST ___________________

LUNCH ___________________

SNACKS ___________________

DINNER ___________________

NOTES

____

____

____

____

WEEKLY MEAL PLANNER

MONDAY

BREAKFAST __________
LUNCH __________
SNACKS __________
DINNER __________

TUESDAY

BREAKFAST __________
LUNCH __________
SNACKS __________
DINNER __________

WEDNESDAY

BREAKFAST __________
LUNCH __________
SNACKS __________
DINNER __________

THURSDAY

BREAKFAST __________
LUNCH __________
SNACKS __________
DINNER __________

FRIDAY

BREAKFAST __________
LUNCH __________
SNACKS __________
DINNER __________

SATURDAY

BREAKFAST __________
LUNCH __________
SNACKS __________
DINNER __________

SUNDAY

BREAKFAST __________
LUNCH __________
SNACKS __________
DINNER __________

NOTES

____
____
____
____

WEEKLY MEAL PLANNER

MONDAY

BREAKFAST ___________________
LUNCH ___________________
SNACKS ___________________
DINNER ___________________

TUESDAY

BREAKFAST ___________________
LUNCH ___________________
SNACKS ___________________
DINNER ___________________

WEDNESDAY

BREAKFAST ___________________
LUNCH ___________________
SNACKS ___________________
DINNER ___________________

THURSDAY

BREAKFAST ___________________
LUNCH ___________________
SNACKS ___________________
DINNER ___________________

FRIDAY

BREAKFAST ___________________
LUNCH ___________________
SNACKS ___________________
DINNER ___________________

SATURDAY

BREAKFAST ___________________
LUNCH ___________________
SNACKS ___________________
DINNER ___________________

SUNDAY

BREAKFAST ___________________
LUNCH ___________________
SNACKS ___________________
DINNER ___________________

NOTES

____
____
____
____

WEEKLY MEAL PLANNER

MONDAY

BREAKFAST ___________________

LUNCH ___________________

SNACKS ___________________

DINNER ___________________

TUESDAY

BREAKFAST ___________________

LUNCH ___________________

SNACKS ___________________

DINNER ___________________

WEDNESDAY

BREAKFAST ___________________

LUNCH ___________________

SNACKS ___________________

DINNER ___________________

THURSDAY

BREAKFAST ___________________

LUNCH ___________________

SNACKS ___________________

DINNER ___________________

FRIDAY

BREAKFAST ___________________

LUNCH ___________________

SNACKS ___________________

DINNER ___________________

SATURDAY

BREAKFAST ___________________

LUNCH ___________________

SNACKS ___________________

DINNER ___________________

SUNDAY

BREAKFAST ___________________

LUNCH ___________________

SNACKS ___________________

DINNER ___________________

NOTES

____

____

____

____

WEEKLY MEAL PLANNER

MONDAY

BREAKFAST ______________________
LUNCH ______________________
SNACKS ______________________
DINNER ______________________

TUESDAY

BREAKFAST ______________________
LUNCH ______________________
SNACKS ______________________
DINNER ______________________

WEDNESDAY

BREAKFAST ______________________
LUNCH ______________________
SNACKS ______________________
DINNER ______________________

THURSDAY

BREAKFAST ______________________
LUNCH ______________________
SNACKS ______________________
DINNER ______________________

FRIDAY

BREAKFAST ______________________
LUNCH ______________________
SNACKS ______________________
DINNER ______________________

SATURDAY

BREAKFAST ______________________
LUNCH ______________________
SNACKS ______________________
DINNER ______________________

SUNDAY

BREAKFAST ______________________
LUNCH ______________________
SNACKS ______________________
DINNER ______________________

NOTES

____
____
____
____

WEEKLY MEAL PLANNER

MONDAY

BREAKFAST ___________________

LUNCH ___________________

SNACKS ___________________

DINNER ___________________

TUESDAY

BREAKFAST ___________________

LUNCH ___________________

SNACKS ___________________

DINNER ___________________

WEDNESDAY

BREAKFAST ___________________

LUNCH ___________________

SNACKS ___________________

DINNER ___________________

THURSDAY

BREAKFAST ___________________

LUNCH ___________________

SNACKS ___________________

DINNER ___________________

FRIDAY

BREAKFAST ___________________

LUNCH ___________________

SNACKS ___________________

DINNER ___________________

SATURDAY

BREAKFAST ___________________

LUNCH ___________________

SNACKS ___________________

DINNER ___________________

SUNDAY

BREAKFAST ___________________

LUNCH ___________________

SNACKS ___________________

DINNER ___________________

NOTES

____

____

____

____

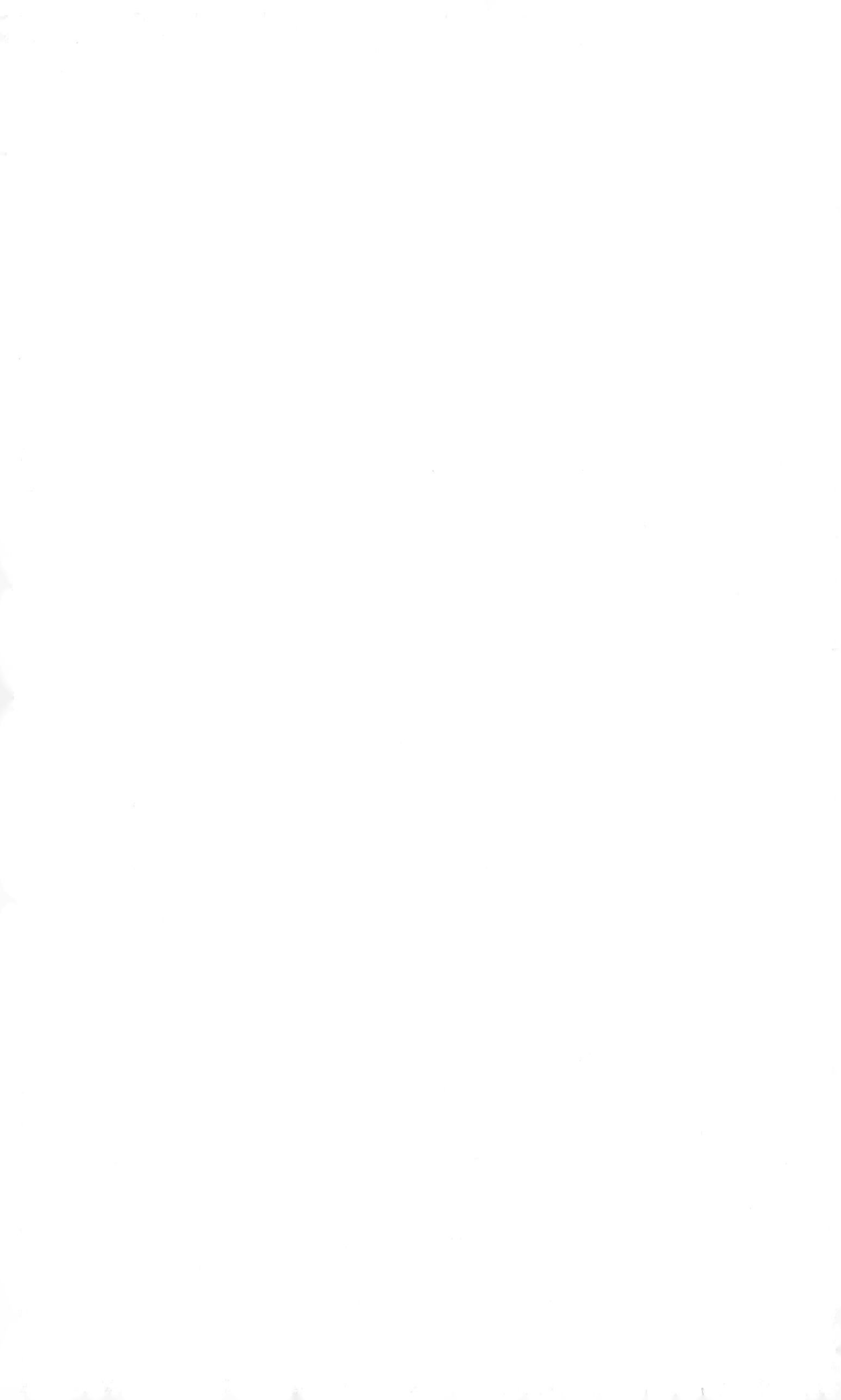

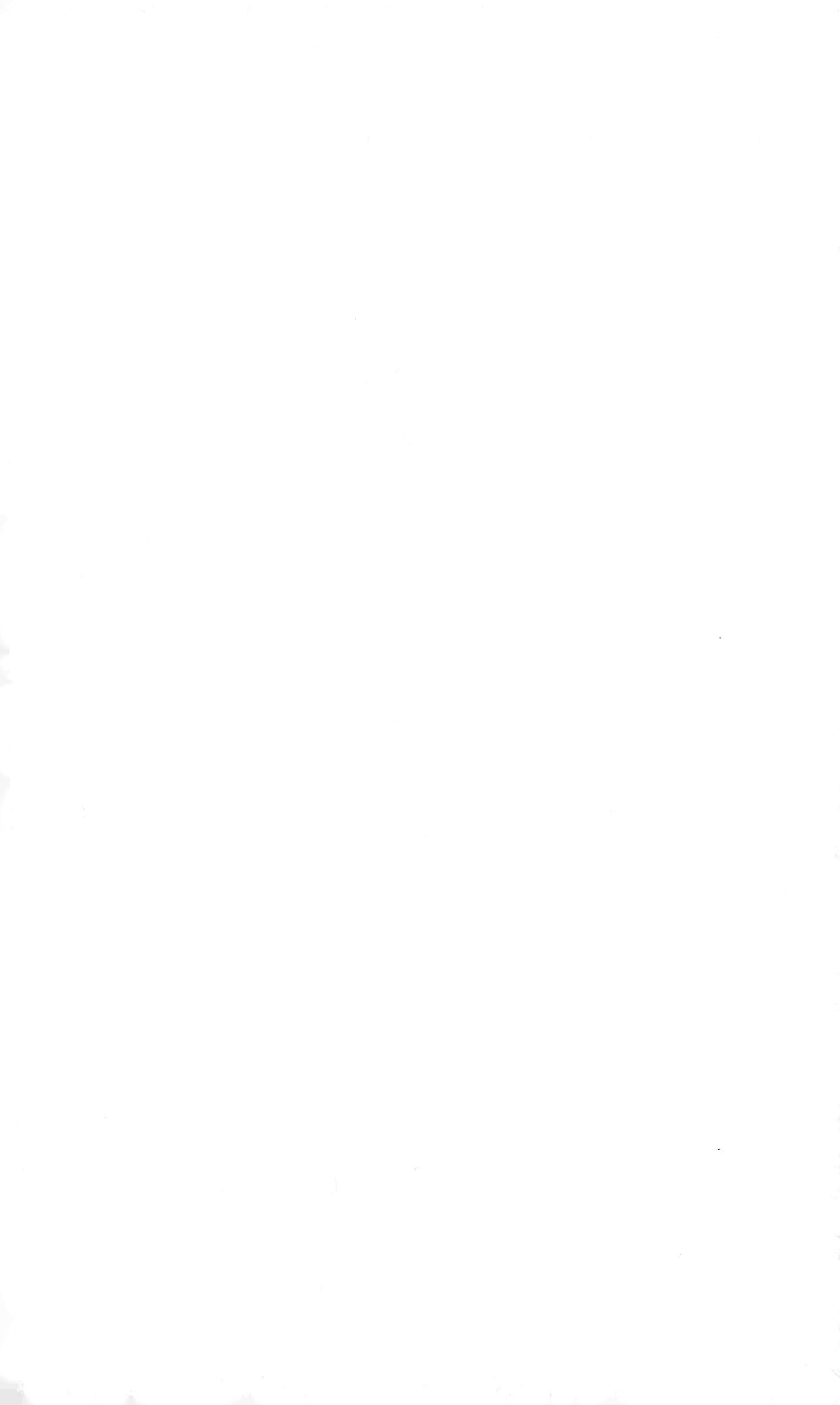